Mastering the DRCOG

Dedication

This book was completed as a result of the unceasing inspiration, encouragement, love and patience that I received from my partner, Dr Clash Ryden, and to the example of my mother, who demonstrated to me throughout life how to put one's mind to a task and achieve it.

Mastering the DRCOG

Jamila Groves
General Practitioner,
Honor Oak Group Practice, Lewisham, London, UK
Belgrave Medical Centre, Westminster, London, UK

Consultant Editors
Lesley Bacon
Consultant in Community Sexual & Reproductive Health,
Lewisham Primary Care Trust, London, UK

Ruth Cochrane
Consultant Obstetrician,
University Hospital Lewisham, London, UK

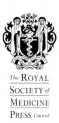

The ROYAL
SOCIETY of
MEDICINE
PRESS Limited

© 2010 Royal Society of Medicine Press Ltd

Published by the Royal Society of Medicine Press Ltd
1 Wimpole Street, London W1G 0AE, UK
Tel: +44 (0)20 7290 2921
Fax: +44 (0)20 7290 2929
Email: publishing@rsm.ac.uk
Website: www.rsmpress.co.uk

British Library Cataloguing in Publication Data
A catalogue record for this book is available from the British Library

ISBN 978-1-85315-827-8

Distribution in Europe and Rest of World:
Marston Book Services Ltd
PO Box 269
Abingdon
Oxon OX14 4YN, UK
Tel: +44 (0)1235 465500
Fax: +44 (0)1235 465555
Email: direct.order@marston.co.uk

Distribution in the USA and Canada:
Royal Society of Medicine Press Ltd
c/o BookMasters Inc.
30 Amberwood Parkway
Ashland, OH 44805, USA
Tel: +1 800 247 6553/+1 800 266 5564
Fax: +1 419 281 6883
Email: orders@bookmasters.com

Distribution in Australia and New Zealand:
Elsevier Australia
30–52 Smidmore Street
Marrickville, NSW 2204, Australia
Tel: +61 2 9517 8999
Fax: +61 2 9517 2249
Email: service@elsevier.com.au

Editorial and typesetting services by B.A. & G.M. Haddock, Ford, Midlothian
Printed and bound in Great Britain by Bell & Bain Ltd, Glasgow

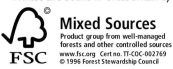

Contents

Preface

In preparing *Mastering the DRCOG*, I have chosen to present information in a way that directly addresses your learning needs as you prepare for the Diploma examination of the Royal College of Obstetricians and Gynaecologists. I have tailored the book around the syllabus so as to equip you with all the information you need in order to pass the DRCOG examination, first time around, and to pass it well.

Essentially, I am writing for medical practitioners who are undergoing specialist training in general practice; doctors who intend to provide primary obstetric and gynaecological care in the UK. However, pioneering medical students and nurse specialists will also find this book invaluable, both as a reference book and for learning, as will doctors working outside the UK. By gaining the Diploma award, you will have the bonus of securing a valuable certification; an achievement that is not easy, but certainly well worthwhile and highly respected. With the diploma award will come the knowledge and confidence required to practice safely and effectively, looking after women and their special needs within the primary care setting.

This book contains a healthy mix of facts, figures and references, presented simply and clearly, in a way that is designed to facilitate your learning. I have used tables to simplify data wherever feasible, and to make facts as digestible as possible to help you learn, as well as make it easy for you to look things up quickly during a consultation. Simple line diagrams are used throughout, so as to explain pictorially the principles that perhaps before confounded you. I find that pictures are also great when explaining concepts to patients, who are genuinely appreciative of the time you take to explain their body to them.

The DRCOG award, being an undoubtedly worthwhile achievement, in such an interesting, challenging and changing area of medicine, made it a real joy for me to prepare for, and I want you to pass it too. The syllabus has both breadth and depth but, at the same time, does not go into unnecessary specialist detail. It is down-to-earth and practical. Working as a full-time NHS GP in London, I have found that having the DRCOG, and the understanding of gynaecology and obstetrics that comes with the certification, absolutely invaluable. Having the DRCOG is useful proof of competence when applying for jobs (whether that be salaried GP posts, partnerships, locums, staff grade hospital appointments, or community women's health clinics). DRCOG certification may allow you to work as a GPwSI (GP with specialist interest) depending on local need, or to enter the private sector. You may be able to run a fertility, or heavy menstrual bleeding, clinic for your area. There are so many opportunities available to you with this award, and such a high and constant need for well trained doctors, that there is nothing possible that you can loose by taking this step.

I very much hope that my excitement for the subject is shared with you as you make your way through these pages, and that on gaining the DRCOG, by reading my book, many a door is opened to you! I wish you all the very best and happy reading!

JAMILA GROVES

About the authors

Dr Jamila Groves MRCGP MBBS BSc DRCOG DFSRH

GENERAL PRACTITIONER

Honor Oak Group Practice, 20 Turnham Road, Lewisham, London SE4 2LA, UK
Belgrave Medical Centre, 13 Pimlico Road, Westminster, London SW1W 8NA, UK
E-mail: jamila.groves@ukdoctor.org

Jamila studied molecular biology in Durham, then medicine at University College London. She was part of the General Practice Vocational Training Scheme of South London, completing the scheme in 2008. Her training was interspersed throughout with travel, and she worked for extended periods in Jamaica, India and China. In these countries, she was involved in rural projects, all of which pioneered female education and health awareness. Jamila has been a salaried GP in inner London for 2 years, and enjoys it immensely, working part-time in Westminster and part-time in Lewisham. She runs women's health clinics which provide antenatal and postpartum care, IUD insertion, menopause management, STI treatment and testing. She has a particular interest in providing care to vulnerable and refugee women and their babies, and in postgraduate education.

Dr Lesley Bacon FFSRH MRCGP

CONSULTANT IN COMMUNITY SEXUAL AND REPRODUCTIVE HEALTH

Waldron Health Centre, Suite 10, Stanley Street, London SE8 5BG, UK

Lesley qualified in medicine from Cambridge and University Hospital London, and then trained as a GP in Scotland (including a year at the Simpson Memorial Maternity Pavilion in Edinburgh, where meticulous audit was promoted long before it became generally fashionable). She then worked for 3 years in Ghana, which profoundly influenced her approach to medicine and to much else. On returning to the UK, she worked in general practice, family planning (as it then was) and genito-urinary medicine, and became convinced that the large areas of overlap between these specialties needed an integrated approach to their development.

She has been a consultant in Sexual and Reproductive Health in SE London since 1996, and is now the lead clinician in Lewisham, which is one of the largest services in the UK, has one of the highest rates of screening for the National Chlamydia Screening Programme and helped to pioneer the supply of oral emergency contraception by community pharmacists. She is a fellow of the Faculty of Sexual and Reproductive Healthcare, has been an examiner for the MFSRH and represents the Faculty on the National Chlamydia Screening Advisory Group. She has contributed to the development of the on-line component of the new DFSRH, and is involved in the training of sexual and reproductive health specialists, GPs, gynaecologists, nurses and pharmacists.

Mrs Ruth Cochrane FRCOG PhD

CONSULTANT OBSTETRICIAN

University Hospital Lewisham, Lewisham High Street, London SE13 6LH, UK

Ruth qualified from the University of Wales in 1981, and became a Consultant of Obstetrics and Gynaecology at University Hospital Lewisham in 1997 where she has been the Lead in GP education for many years. Ruth is a role model for GP Specialist Trainees, training many young doctors every year. Dedicated to her job, her patients, and to excellence, Ruth has been a Fellow of the Royal College of Obstetricians and Gynaecologists since 2003. Her special interests include the management of fibroids, recurrent pregnancy loss, and high-risk obstetrics as well as undergraduate and postgraduate teaching.

INTRODUCTION

This book is written with two main aims: to help you pass the Diploma of the Royal College of Obstetricians and Gynaecologists (DRCOG), and to make to you competent and confident in the management of women and their reproductive or sexual problems within the primary care setting. This book will prepare you for the care of the simple, yet common, daily difficulties encountered by women and those which present to the General Practitioner (GP) time and time again. The book covers which pill is the best for acne, the treatment options for heavy periods and the mechanism of a normal vaginal delivery to name but a few topics. This book also aims to equip the reader with emergency essentials such as how to resuscitate a new born baby, when to refer rapidly to a suspected cancer clinic, and how to manage a woman who has just been raped.

The book is organised to reflect and fulfil the syllabus for the DRCOG examination directly, and chapters are laid out exactly to follow the DRCOG syllabus format.

The current DRCOG syllabus can be found on the Royal College of Obstetricians and Gynaecologists website – <http://www.rcog.org.uk/index.asp?PageID=1977>.

The following paragraphs written in italics and within speech marks are the syllabus, quoted word for word for your convenience:

'The DRCOG examination is an assessment of knowledge and competence in the subjects of obstetrics, gynaecology, sexual health and family planning.'

'It should be clearly understood by candidates that the DRCOG examination will assess knowledge and clinical problem-solving skills in the above domains as applied to Women's health at a level appropriate for a General Practitioner (GP) in the United Kingdom.'

MODULE 1: BASIC CLINICAL SKILLS

'You will be expected to understand the patterns of symptoms in patients presenting with obstetric problems, gynaecological problems, sexually transmitted infections and patients in a family planning setting.'

'You will be expected to demonstrate an understanding of the pathophysiological basis of physical signs and understand the indications, risks, benefits and effectiveness of investigations in a clinical setting.'

'You will be required to demonstrate an understanding of the components of effective verbal and non-verbal communication.'

'You will need to be aware of relevant ethical and legal issues including the implications of the legal status of the unborn child, the legal issues relating to medical certification and issues related to medical confidentiality.'

Module 1 covers all the basic clinical skills required of a GP in the UK. Most of the skills will have been learnt in medical school and re-enforced and practiced while working as a junior doctor. However, this book will not assume any particular prior knowledge, and is written in a clear style that should be accessible and understandable to the medical student, as well as to those doctors who have perhaps been out of practice for some time.

MODULE 2: BASIC SURGICAL SKILLS

'You will be expected to demonstrate an understanding of commonly performed obstetric and gynaecological surgical procedures including their complications.'

'You will need to be aware of commonly encountered infections, including an understanding of the principles of infection control.'

'You will be expected to interpret pre-operative investigations and be aware of the principles involved in appropriate pre-operative and post-operative care.'

'You will be expected to understand the legal issues surrounding consent in all clinical situations including termination of pregnancy.'

Module 2 looks at the surgical treatment for women with gynaecological complaints. The information is presented at a level suitable for a gynaecology specialist trainee, and provides excellent insight for GPs who have not done a gynaecology job. This chapter is not intended to teach doctors how to operate, but rather to understand surgical procedures so that accurate information can be given to patients, both before and after surgical treatment.

Topics covered in this chapter will include hysteroscopy, total and subtotal hysterectomy, myomectomy, and prolapse repair. Mention will be made regarding infection control, and the risks and benefits of the different surgical procedures.

MODULE 3: ANTENATAL CARE

'You will be expected to understand and demonstrate appropriate knowledge and attitudes in relation to peri-conceptional care, antenatal care and maternal complications of pregnancy.'

'An awareness of substance misuse, psychiatric illness, problems of pregnancy at extremes of reproductive age and of domestic violence in relation to pregnancy is expected. An appreciation of emotional issues and cultural awareness is expected.'

'You will be expected to have a good understanding of common medical disorders and the effect that pregnancy may have on them, and also their effect, in turn, upon the pregnancy. A knowledge of therapeutics in antenatal care is expected. You will be expected to demonstrate your ability to assess and manage these conditions.'

'You will be expected to understand the principles of antenatal screening including screening for structural defects, chromosomal abnormalities and haemoglobinopathies and the effects upon fetus and neonate of relevant infections during pregnancy. You will need to show understanding of the roles of other professionals, the importance of liaison and empathic teamwork.'

Module 3 is an important chapter. It explains thoroughly the care of pregnant women, from the time a couple presents for advice concerning conception, to confirming the pregnancy, routine scans and tests that are recommended, and how to manage pregnancies with complications. There is a lot of advice on the minor upsets that are common during pregnancy, and tips of simple ways to help. The interlinking roles of the midwives, GPs, obstetricians, the woman and her family are discussed.

MODULE 4: MANAGEMENT OF LABOUR AND DELIVERY

'You will be expected to have the knowledge, understanding and judgement to be capable of initial management of intrapartum problems in a hospital and in a community setting. This will include: knowledge and understanding of normal and abnormal labour, data and investigation interpretation, induction and augmentation of labour, assessment of fetal wellbeing and compromise.'

'An understanding of the management of all obstetric emergencies is expected.'

'You will need to demonstrate appropriate knowledge of regional anaesthesia, analgesia and operative delivery including caesarean section.'

'You will need to be able to demonstrate respect for cultural and religious differences in attitudes to childbirth.'

Module 4 is regarding delivery of the fetus, and the transition of the pregnant woman into motherhood. The normal vaginal delivery is explained, and there are ample diagrams to help visualise this. Difficult and obstructed labours are explained in a way that an obstetric specialist trainee would be able to manage emergencies, and a GP would able to understand what goes on behind the doors of labour ward. It is important to have this understanding in order to be able to explain things to new mothers and their support networks confidently. Often, many questions arise only once things have settled down, and the new mother is back at home.

MODULE 5: POST-PARTUM AND NEONATAL PROBLEMS

'You will be expected to understand and demonstrate appropriate knowledge, management skills and attitudes in relation to postpartum maternal problems including: the normal and abnormal postpartum period, postpartum haemorrhage, therapeutics, perineal care, psychological disorders, infant feeding and breast problems.'

'You will be expected to demonstrate an understanding of the investigation and management of immediate neonatal problems including neonatal resuscitation.'

Module 5 focuses on the newborn baby and the new mother both of whom are recovering from delivery. It provides practical advice and tips on how to succeed in breast-feeding, and how best to provide support for the new mother and her family. Important neonatal problems are explained as well as the important post-natal problems that can arise.

MODULE 6: GYNAECOLOGICAL PROBLEMS

'You will be expected to demonstrate appropriate knowledge, management skills and attitudes in relation to benign gynaecological problems including: urogynaecology, paediatric and adolescent gynaecology, endocrine problems, pelvic pain and abnormal vaginal bleeding. This will include knowledge of early pregnancy loss, including clinical features, investigation and management of disorders leading to early pregnancy loss: miscarriage (including recurrent), ectopic pregnancy and molar pregnancy.'

'You will be expected to demonstrate an ability to assess and manage common sexually transmitted infections including HIV/AIDS and be familiar with their modes of transmission and clinical features. You will be expected to understand the principles of contact tracing.'

'You will also be expected to know the basis of national screening programmes and their local implementation through local care pathways. You will be expected to demonstrate appropriate knowledge of clinical features, investigation and management of pre-malignant and malignant conditions of the female genital tract. You will be expected to have an understanding of the indications and limitations of screening for pre-malignant and malignant disease. An understanding of the options available for palliative and terminal care including relief of symptoms and community support will be expected.'

This module attempts to cover the vast speciality of gynaecology. Sexually transmitted infections and the cervical screening programme make up a large part of this module. Management of miscarriage, including recurrent miscarriage, and the aetiology and management options for ectopic pregnancy are also covered at some length, as are the problems of uterine prolapse and polycystic ovarian syndrome.

MODULE 7: FERTILITY CONTROL

'The examiners will expect you to demonstrate appropriate knowledge and attitudes in relation to sub-fertility. This includes an understanding of the epidemiology, aetiology, management and prognosis of male and female fertility problems. You will be expected to have a broad-based knowledge of investigation and management of the infertile couple in a primary care setting and appropriate knowledge of assisted reproductive techniques including and the legal and ethical implications of these procedures.'

'You will be expected to understand the indications, contra-indications, complications, mode of action and efficacy of all reversible and irreversible contraceptive methods.'

'You will be expected to demonstrate appropriate knowledge of abortion and should be familiar with the accompanying laws related to abortion, consent, child protection and the Sexual Offences Act(s). You will be expected to demonstrate appropriate knowledge, management skills and attitudes in relation to fertility control and termination of pregnancy. There may be conscientious objection to the acquisition of certain skills in areas of sexual and reproductive health but knowledge and appropriate attitudes as described above will be expected.'

Module 7 explains and clarifies the uncomfortable and troubling condition of subfertility, as well as unwanted fertility (birth control). All contraceptive methods available in the UK are described, and the benefits for each method outlined. When unwanted pregnancy occurs, the option of terminating the pregnancy is open to women in the UK. Because of this, the methods used to terminate pregnancies are explained, as well as the laws that govern abortion.

MODULE 8: Material that is not contained within the DRCOG syllabus

We have written an extra chapter for you, which we feel is valuable in many ways. Although this chapter contains information that is not requested for the DRCOG examination, these topics are highly relevant to any doctor working in the field of women's health. Module 8 covers controversial issues which should you not have come across in work or personal experience as yet, you almost certainly will do so in the near future. Women are often treated differently to men in society; this can be appropriate and necessary, but may be unwelcome, discriminatory and hurtful causing morbidity, which presents to the GP.

Module 1:
Basic clinical skills

You will be expected to understand the patterns of symptoms in patients presenting with obstetric problems, gynaecological problems, sexually transmitted infections and patients in a family planning setting.

You will be expected to demonstrate an understanding of the pathophysiological basis of physical signs and understand the indications, risks, benefits and effectiveness of investigations in a clinical setting.

You will be required to demonstrate an understanding of the components of effective verbal and non-verbal communication.

You will need to be aware of relevant ethical and legal issues including the implications of the legal status of the unborn child, the legal issues relating to medical certification and issues related to medical confidentiality.

THE WOMAN PRESENTING TO THE GP

Women present to their GPs with all sorts of complaints, and a great many of these relate to symptoms they feel, or concerns they have, regarding their reproductive organs. This chapter covers the main symptoms that women present with, and explains how a GP should go about dealing with them. You may find that such work feels very different from dealing with the same problems in hospital; you will be looking at the medical problem in a much wider context and there are a great many more uncertainties to be managed.

BASIC ANATOMY

The female reproductive anatomy is composed of external and internal structures, all of which are difficult for women to view themselves. Most women can only see their own external genitalia with the aid of a mirror, and the internal genitalia are only visible with the aid of instrumentation by a second party. Because the female genitalia are concealed in this way, difficulties can occur as examination by a doctor can be perceived to be a bit too intrusive, making women reluctant to present. This makes it quite easy for abnormalities such as genital warts or painless ulcers to go unnoticed by a woman for some time. However, many women (and indeed men) feel that the compact and subtle design of the female reproductive system is a clear artistic advantage when compared to what may be described as candour of the male.

EXTERNAL GENITALIA

The pudendum is the term given to the external genitalia of the female (Fig. 1.1); it comes from the Latin *pudere*, to be ashamed. The vulva is the term given to the labial opening to the vagina.

The two larger (major) labia (lips) are fatty skin folds that form the perimeter of the vulva. In the adult female, their outside surface is covered with pubic hair. The labia majora lie over two smaller labia minora. The introitus is the term given to the opening of the vagina; it comes from the Latin *intro*, meaning within. The vaginal introitus lies posterior to the opening of the urethra in the vestibule. The labia minora meet in the mid-line anteriorly to form a hood over the clitoris. The clitoris is a small mass of erectile tissue situated at the anterior apex of the vestibule. It is a highly sensitive area, important for sexual arousal and stimulation of this area leads to orgasm. It is homologous to the penis of the male. The perineum is the area of skin and connective tissue that lies between the vulva and the anus.

INTERNAL GENITALIA

The vagina is the muscular canal that runs from the introitus to the uterine cervix. The term vagina is the Latin word for scabbard (the sheath for the blade of a sword or dagger), the sword in this context seemingly refers to a penis (Fig. 1.2).

The uterus is the child-bearing organ of the female reproductive tract. It is composed of the uterine fundus (the part of a hollow organ furthest from the opening), uterine corpus (body) and uterine cervix (neck). The uterine wall is composed of a muscular outer layer known as the myometrium, and a secretory inner layer known as the endometrium. The tissue that makes up the endometrium is shed each month in response to the hormonal changes of the menstrual cycle.

The fallopian tubes extend from the uterine fundus to the ovaries on either side. The lumens of the tubes are lined

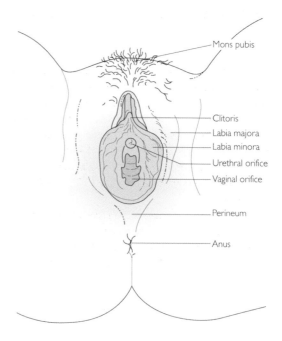

Figure 1.1 External genitalia.

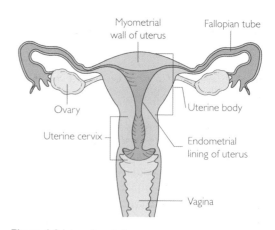

Figure 1.2 Internal genitalia.

with cilia; it is due to the peristaltic action of these that the ovum or embryo is transported down into the uterine cavity. Each fallopian tube opens into the peritoneum with fronds known as fimbriae which act to catch the ovum at ovulation.

The ovary is the female gonad, where all of the female gametes (ova) are stored. There is one ovary, each about the size of an almond, suspended at the end of each fallopian tube by the ovarian ligament. Each ovary is attached to the uterus by the broad ligament. As well as being the female gonad, the ovary also acts as an endocrine organ, producing a number of hormones, including oestrogen.

The areas in the pelvis lateral to the uterus (where the fallopian tubes and ovaries lie) are known as the left and right adnexa.

BASIC PHYSIOLOGY: THE MENSTRUAL CYCLE

MENSTRUATION

The first day of the menstrual cycle is taken to be the first day of flow of menstrual blood. The blood loss is obvious to the woman, and can easily be used as a landmark that she can record and remember. Menstruation is the result of desquamation of the endometrium. Necrotic endometrial tissue is shed along with blood and fibrinolysin which prevents clotting and thus allows the lost tissue to flow easily from the body. There is also an accompanying outflow of leukocytes which makes the uterus highly resistant to infection during menstruation even though the endometrial surfaces are denuded. This is of great protective value.

Menstruation is usually slightly painful, and this is normal. The pain is due to the natural local release of prostaglandins during menstruation. The prostaglandins have a useful role in that they cause contractions of the myometrium, which are required to expel the tissue and blood from the uterine cavity. Some women are more sensitive to prostaglandins than others, and some women produce more prostaglandins than others making periods rather more painful, but the pain should be bearable with simple analgesia such as ibuprofen or paracetamol. When periods are unbearably painful (dysmenorrhoea) or heavy (menorrhagia), this is not normal and will be discussed in later chapters.

The subsequent events of the menstrual cycle are much more discrete and most women are unaware of the complexities going on inside them at the different times of the month (Fig. 1.3).

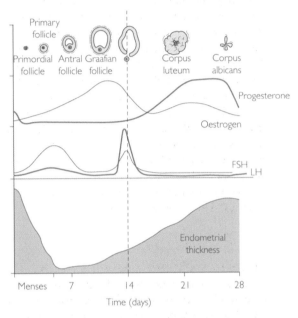

Figure 1.3 Menstrual cycle.

Follicle stimulating hormone and growth of the follicle

Follicle stimulating hormone (FSH) begins to be released from the anterior pituitary gland during the first couple of days of the menstrual cycle, blood levels peaking on the third, fourth and fifth days of menstruation.

FSH, as its name suggests, stimulates growth of the ovarian follicles. In fact, 6–12 primordial follicles are stimulated by the action of FSH every cycle. The ova within these follicles enlarge, the granulosa cells that surround them grow in both size and number, and fluid accumulates to form what are known as antral follicles.

Oestrogen and further growth of one of the follicles

Over the next few days, the granulosa cells produce increasing amounts of oestrogen as they continue to grow and divide. After one week of growth, one of the follicles will have outgrown all of the others which therefore involute and die (Fig. 1.4).

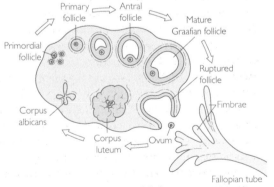

Figure 1.4 Ovary and ovarian follicle.

Oestrogen acts via a positive feedback system on the remaining antral follicle, stimulating an explosive rate of growth, as well as a surge of oestrogen production. The mature follicle that results is known as the Graafian follicle. It is approximately 15 mm in diameter, and stretches the ovarian wall, disfiguring it to allow it to be just visible to an ultrasonographer. Once the Graafian follicle is mature, oestrogen production reaches a critical level which triggers receptors in the hypothalamus.

Ovulation

At this point, the hypothalamus secretes increased gonadotrophin releasing hormone (GnRH) which, in turn, stimulates the release of luteinizing hormone (LH) and FSH from the anterior pituitary gland in rapidly increasing quantity. LH and FSH act synergistically on the mature follicle, causing it to swell. The granulosa cells of the follicle cease their oestrogen production, and switch to making progesterone. The capsule of the follicle releases proteolytic enzymes that weaken the ovarian wall, and this, combined with the pressure of the swollen follicle, causes the wall of the ovary that overlies the follicle to perforate. The ovum is then expelled energetically from the follicle and ovary in what is known as ovulation. The ovum lands on the fimbriae of the fallopian tubes, and is then wafted by the rhythmic movements of the cilia down into the tubular lumen.

Ovulation is felt by some women as a sharp pain in one of the iliac fossae, and may be accompanied by a light watery discharge. Both of these symptoms are normal, not indicating any pathology. The pain is known as Mittelschmerz pain (derived from *Mittel*, the German word for middle, and *Schmerz* meaning pain), and can be treated with simple analgesia such as paracetamol if necessary.

The corpus luteum

In the hours following ovulation, the granulosa cells of the follicle change rapidly; they enlarge to become three times their original size and becomes lipid filled. This clump of cells gains a yellow tinge due to the high lipid content, and is referred to as the corpus luteum, from the Latin yellow body. The corpus luteum is extremely important; it secretes a copious amount of progesterone for its small size, along with some oestrogen and, by so doing, sustains the endometrium making it secretory and inviting to a fertilized egg. The corpus luteum hold this role for 12 days, and then involutes and dies. If fertilization did not occur, the progesterone and oestrogen levels drop swiftly with the death of the corpus luteum, the endometrium is no longer sustained, and is shed as menstruation as the cycle begins once again.

TAKING A GYNAECOLOGICAL HISTORY

The first step is to take a clear history, first allowing the woman to explain her symptoms in her own words, and then moving onto more directed questions to help hone down on the problem. Most problems will present as pain, vaginal discharge, vaginal bleeding, or fertility issues such as contraception, assisted conception, and pregnancy.

It is important that a doctor is able to elicit what the woman worried about accurately. This is achieved by asking about:

- *Symptomatology*: what, when, where, why.
- *Menstrual cycle*: length, regularity, pain, heaviness.
- *Contraception*: past, present, under consideration for future use.
- *Gravidity and parity*: miscarriages, terminations, ectopics, deliveries, obstetric complications.
- *Sexual partners*: regular or casual, protected or unprotected, casual or considered, number of partners, gender of partners, any partners of high HIV risk.
- *Previous gynaecological treatments, operations or problems*: colposcopy, pelvic inflammatory disease, endometriosis, ovarian cysts, recurrent thrush or urinary infections.
- *Any other issues*.

It is important that the woman herself is allowed to lead the consultation by discussing what she feels is important.

GOOD PRACTICE POINTS 1.1–1.3

• When taking a gynaecological history be aware that there may be unrecognised mental health problems, undisclosed domestic violence, hidden psychosexual issues, or other secret agendas underlying symptoms.

• Do not insist on history taking if you sense resistance and feel unable to secure the woman's confidence. It usually helps if you explain why you need the information, but remember that sometimes trust is not assumed but will need to be earned by a GP over a series of visits.

• Remember that it is the patient who defines the problem, not the doctor (Ian McWhinney, 1997, in *A Textbook of Family Medicine*), and that however pushed for time the doctor may be, authoritarian consulting styles tend not to work. (David Pendleton, Schofield, Tate & Havelock, 2003, in the *New Consultation*).

EXAMINING THE FEMALE PATIENT

EXAMINATION ENVIRONMENT

All patients should be treated with dignity and respect by their doctor during examination. Due care is of particular importance when a gynaecological examination is being performed, as this involves looking at an extremely private area of the body, both for the woman herself and for her partner. Insensitive examination can cause long-lasting distress to the woman and have an emotional impact that is not easily alleviated. For these reasons, a woman should undress only when behind a curtain, and should be provided with disposable paper towelling with which she can cover her pelvic area to allow her a sense of control and privacy when lying on the examination couch.

A chaperone should always be offered when performing an intimate examination; if a chaperone is not available, the woman should be offered an opportunity to return for examination when a chaperone will be available. If a chaperone is declined, this should be documented in the medical notes.

INSPECTION

When performing a gynaecological examination, the first thing to be carried out is an inspection of the external genitalia for any abnormalities. This is most easily done with the woman lying in the lithotomy position (on her back, with her legs flexed at the knees and feet flat on the examination couch, or in stirrups).

The labia, mons pubis, and inner thighs should be examined for the presence of any unusual lumps, rashes, ulcers or any other abnormality. Any tattoos or genital piercings should be noted. If a rash or itch is present, there should be a detailed look at the pubic hairs searching for any evidence for pubic lice or scabies. Shaving the public hairs may have resulted in in-growing hairs, septic spots, or rashes. Especially in overweight women, candidal rashes may develop in the inguinal–labial folds. Bruising or abrasions may be the sign of sexual abuse. Female genital mutilation may have resulted in the absence of some of the genital organs or tightening of the vaginal introitus. A hymen may or may not be visible.

BIMANUAL EXAMINATION

Performing a bimanual examination conventionally takes place with the doctor on the right side of the patient who is lying in lithotomy position, so the right hand palpates the uterus from within the vagina, and the left hand palpates the uterus through the abdominal wall. To achieve this, the doctor places the index and middle finger of the right hand into the posterior fornix of the vagina (behind the cervix). Gentle pressure is applied to lift the uterus anteriorly towards the left hand on the abdomen. The right and left adnexa are palpated in a similar way, by moving the fingers to the right and left of the cervix, while the left hand moves to the right and left iliac fossae (Fig. 1.5).

A bimanual examination is a good way of estimating the size and shape of the uterus, to determine whether there are any masses in the pelvis, and to assess absence or presence of pelvic pain. The non-pregnant uterus is about the size of a chicken egg; a uterus at 8 weeks' gestation is about the size of a small orange, and at 12 weeks' gestation about the size of a grapefruit. At 12 weeks' gestation, the uterus is just palpable in the abdomen as it manages to project its fundus above the symphysis pubis. The uterus can be enlarged for reasons other than pregnancy, such as the presence of uterine fibroids.

Assessing the position of the uterus within the pelvis is another important reason for carrying out a bimanual examination. Sources vary, but the consensus is that approximately 80% of women have an anteverted uterus, with the uterine fundus lying anteriorly over the bladder, and 20% of women have a retroverted uterus, with the uterine fundus pointing posteriorly towards the sacrum. These positions are normal anatomical variants with no significance with regards to fertility. Some women with a retroverted uterus feel deep dyspareunia, and changing of sexual position can successfully alleviate this. The significance of uterine position

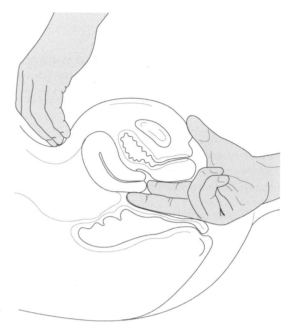

Figure 1.5 Bimanual examination.

is important to healthcare professionals when inserting a coil or doing any surgical procedure that involves blind instrumentation of the uterine cavity, such as dilatation and curettage, or termination of pregnancy.

Pain during bimanual examination is another sign of pelvic pathology. A bimanual examination when performed correctly on a healthy woman may be slightly uncomfortable, but should be painless. If there is pain on touching the cervix, this is known as cervical excitation, and is often a sign of a sexually transmitted infection or an ectopic pregnancy. Pain elicited on palpation of the adnexa is known as adnexal tenderness. This, again, may be a sign of a sexually transmitted infection or ectopic pregnancy, or may be due to the presence of endometriosis, or some sort of ovarian pathology such as a dermoid cyst.

SPECULUM EXAMINATION

Having inspected the external genitalia, with consent, a Cusco speculum (Fig. 1.6) should be inserted into the vagina and opened gently. This allows viewing of the vaginal walls and cervix. All speculums used in the UK should now be for single-use only. Lubricant can be applied to the speculum prior to insertion if the vagina is dry, the exception to this is that should you be taking cervical cytology lubricant must not be used, but rather warm water.

Should there be uterine prolapse, this is often easily identified on examination with the Cusco speculum as the cervix will be seen to be lying rather low within the vagina. However, for examination of suspected vaginal wall prolapse, a Sims speculum is often preferred. Use of this speculum requires the woman to lie on her left side, with her left knee flexed against the abdomen and the right knee flexed and raised slightly, often by resting the right foot on the wall.

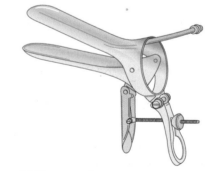

Figure 1.6 Cusco speculum.

GOOD PRACTICE POINT 1.4

- Make sure you have a selection of different sized speculums available as you may find it impossible to view the cervix if the speculum is of incorrect size.

NORMAL PHYSIOLOGICAL VAGINAL DISCHARGE

Women naturally have a vaginal discharge which keeps the vagina acidic and healthy, and provides the lubrication necessary for comfortable coitus. Vaginal discharge increases physiologically around the time of ovulation, and can become quite slippery and wet. This type of discharge usually lasts for only a few days before the discharge becomes thicker, sticky and drier during the second half of the menstrual cycle. A normal vaginal discharge is free of odour and does not itch. The colour ranges from a transparent colourless to a white or slightly yellow tinted shade.

Excluding infectious causes of the discharge

On speculum examination, it is usually possible to gain a good idea as to whether discharge is normal looking or not. However, it is always recommended that a swab for NAAT (the Nucleic Acid Amplification Test) is taken for chlamydia (some laboratories can also use this swab for gonorrhoea testing, but not all) and a charcoal swab is taken for, thrush, bacterial vaginosis, trichomonas and gonorrhoea.

Management of normal physiological discharge

For many women, simple re-assurance that a discharge is normal is all that is required once infectious causes have been ruled out. There is great variety in the quantity of normal vaginal discharge; some women producing more than they would prefer. Excessive vaginal discharge may lead to embarrassment, especially as it can seep through clothes, in which case wearing panty-liners can help. It is important that frequent washing with soap is avoided, as this can exacerbate the problem and cause bacterial vaginosis. The management of physiological discharge is best done in the primary care setting, gynaecological referral being unnecessary unless other pathology is suspected.

INVESTIGATIONS

Patients are often very keen to have investigations done. Everyone is encouraged by the media and pharmaceutical industry to seek out illnesses they may not know they have, and can be made to worry about any small symptom they may experience. Without knowing it, patients may find themselves accessing inaccurate information, or poor research data with no real evidence base. As a result, the conclusions drawn are misconstrued, leading to the development of all sorts of unnecessary feelings of fear and vulnerability. In addition, people do fall ill at times, and become appropriately worried when they do so. These uncomfortable feelings of apprehension are intensified when they do not know what it is that is happening to their bodies. The seemingly logical way forward to them is to seek out some sort of investigation to find out what is wrong.

The GP on the other hand is often not so keen on investigations, and rightly so. Although of great overall benefit to patients and the healthcare system alike, investigations can also do a lot of harm, and GPs should act to protect their patients from this. Screening, for example, comes at a high cost to the healthy. Often things are found incidentally that would never do any harm, but simply knowing that they are there causes anxiety to the patient and doctor alike. Also, the healthy, with very low risk of disease, have to take time from work (or whatever else they do), think about what they are doing (simply having an investigation causes a certain degree of stress in all of us), await results (few of us have patience these days), perhaps be exposed to radiation (particularly high with computed tomography [CT] scans, but still significant with X-rays), or have to expose ourselves (such as with a smear test or trans-vaginal ultrasound scan). The process of undergoing investigation can instil a feeling of powerlessness and dependence that may encourage the development of external loci of control in individuals whom, if the test were not available, would never have to worry.

Then there is the cost. There are incentives in place to ensure that GPs maintain their role as the main gatekeepers of the National Health Service, and keep their investigations (and referrals) to the minimum required in order to reach a diagnosis while still maintaining adequate care for their patients.

So there is a real skill to be learnt here; how to know when no investigations are necessary, and how to communicate this effectively to patients so that they feel genuinely re-assured and, at the same time, to recognise when the benefits of screening outweigh the burden and cost of having it done making the test worthwhile, and when investigations are indisputably necessary or urgent.

PREGNANCY TESTING

Urine pregnancy tests should be available in all GP surgeries. They are quick and simple to perform, and can be carried out by doctors, nurses or healthcare assistants. There are a number of home pregnancy testing kits available for purchase over the counter, but some women find these hard to read or too expensive, so often come to the doctor for testing when the need arises. All doctors should have a low threshold for doing a pregnancy test on any woman of child-bearing age who presents with amenorrhoea, irregular bleeding, lost IUD threads or iliac fossa pain, as well as those with missed periods.

GOOD PRACTICE POINT 1.5

- To be safe, treat all women of child-bearing age as pregnant until proven otherwise. Nearly all gynaecological symptoms in women of child-bearing age can be caused by pregnancy.

BLOOD TESTING

Blood tests are generally necessary if there is a possible hormone imbalance. For example, in a patient with secondary amenorrhoea with no obvious cause, it would be appropriate to request the following blood tests: a full blood count, prolactin, thyroid function tests, LH, FSH, sex hormone binding globulin and testosterone.

If anaemia is suspected, for example in a patient with heavy menstrual bleeding, then a full blood count, along with a ferritin level or iron studies would be appropriate and is recommended by NICE guidance. If the iron levels are found to be low, this would confirm the history of heavy bleeding given by the patient, and gives the doctor an idea the severity of the problem. Remember that ferritin is an acute phase protein, and can be raised for a number of reasons, such as concurrent infection.

FSH and mid-luteal progesterone

Blood tests are useful for the assessment of subfertility. FSH taken on days 3–5 of the menstrual cycle should be less than 20 mIU/ml. If FSH is found to be raised, and particularly should it be over 30 mIU/ml, ovarian failure due to perimenopause or menopause should be suspected. Testing serum FSH levels is useful in confirming the menopause in women on progestogen contraceptive methods that prevent menstruation, such as the intra-uterine system (the Mirena), the subdermal implant or the progestogen-only pill. In women of perimenopausal age, it can often be unclear whether amenorrhoea is due to the contraceptive method, pregnancy, or the menopause. If there have been no periods for 12 months, and serum FSH is raised > 30 mU/mg on two occasions at least 1 month apart, contraception should be continued for another year if the woman is over the age of 50 years, and for 2 years if the woman is under the age of 50 years.

Serum progesterone taken 7 days before the next period is due is a helpful indicator of ovulation. Levels should really be over 23 ng/ml if ovulation has occurred. If there has been no ovulation, or if the test is done at any other time in the menstrual cycle, the level may be < 5 ng/ml.

> ### GOOD PRACTICE POINT 1.6
>
> - Be aware of when in the menstrual cycle blood tests for FSH and progesterone should be taken. This should be on days 3, 4 or 5 of the menstrual cycle for FSH, and 7 days after the predicted ovulation date for progesterone.

Beta-human chorionic gonadotrophin testing

Beta-HCG is a test not often used in the primary care setting. It can be used to diagnose pregnancy on the rare occasions when a woman feels sure that she is pregnant, has had a late period, yet has a negative urine pregnancy test. The beta-HCG test is the definitive test for pregnancy; if this is not raised, the woman can be assured with confidence that she is not pregnant. Beta-HCG is used in secondary care to monitor ectopic pregnancies and the resolution of molar pregnancies (see Module 6).

HIV testing

All pregnant women are tested for HIV when they first see their midwife unless they chose to opt-out. Non-pregnant women may be offered HIV testing if they are thought to be at risk or if they want re-assurance (for example, after the end of a relationship). Women at highest risk of contracting HIV include those who inject drugs, prostitutes, those from the African or south-east Asian subcontinent or the Caribbean, and victims of rape. However, any woman who has been sexually active without a condom may have become HIV positive. Bear in mind that HIV is also passed from mother to child, and the first cohort of HIV-positive babies has now become adult. Before an HIV test, it is good practice to counsel the woman on what it would mean to receive a positive HIV test result, and what could be done for her should that situation arise.

Syphilis testing

All women with genital ulceration should be tested for syphilis, even if clinically the ulcers look typical of herpes simplex.

Rubella testing

All women who are trying to conceive should be tested to ensure that they are immune to rubella infection. Should they lack immunity, the MMR vaccine (measles, mumps and rubella) should be administered before pregnancy (the rubella single-antigen vaccine is no longer available in the UK). If a woman is found to lack immunity to rubella during pregnancy (rubella immunity is done as part of routine antenatal care at the booking appointment), she should be offered the MMR after delivery of the child. Counselling would be recommended should the pregnant mother succumb to rubella during pregnancy (see Module 3).

MICROBIOLOGICAL TESTING

Mid-stream urine

Collection of mid-stream urine (MSU) is important to confirm or exclude the presence of a urinary tract infection (UTI). The woman should be instructed to urinate the first bit of her stream into the toilet, catch some urine 'mid-stream', then let the remainder of the urine fall as normal into the toilet. This has been shown to be the most effective way of catching urine from the bladder without contaminating organisms from the urethra or vulva falling into the sample pot. Collecting an MSU sample can be quite tricky for some women to do, particularly those with weak pelvic floor muscles, obesity, or musculoskeletal problems.

Microscopy, culture and sensitivity (MC&S)

The MSU sample is sent to the microbiology laboratory for microscopy, culture and sensitivity (MC&S). If the laboratory reports the presence of mixed organisms as probable contaminants, it is likely that the woman used poor technique to collect the sample, although she should not be blamed for this. If symptoms persist, a repeat sample should be taken. If the laboratory reports no growth, yet the woman is symptomatic of urinary tract infection, it is possible that she is suffering from a viral urinary tract infection, chlamydial urinary tract infection, or possibly interstitial cystitis. If the MC&S report names an organism as being present, it will also list antibiotics to which the organism is sensitive and resistant. The doctor can then choose an appropriate antibiotic to clear the organism.

GOOD PRACTICE POINTS 1.7–1.8

- Do not forget to ask about adverse drug reactions before prescribing antibiotics, especially penicillins.

- Do not forget to check whether a woman is pregnant or breast feeding before choosing an antibiotic to prescribe.

First-catch urine

Collection of first-catch urine involves catching the urine that is first to pass from the urethral at micturition. This method is used for testing for chlamydia, chosen as this is the most effective way of catching any chlamydial bacteria resident in the urethra. First-catch urine testing is more commonly used for diagnosing Chlamydia in males, but is available as an alternative to vaginal swabbing for females in some areas.

NAATs vaginal swabs for chlamydia

All women having IUD fitting, hysteroscopy, or an abortion should be offered a NAAT chlamydia test prior to their procedure. Most GP surgeries and all sexual health clinics offer free opportunistic screening, as do many universities and some health clubs. Home testing kits can be bought over the counter. In addition to this, most areas in England have a local service for screening young people aged 15–24 years, known as the National Chlamydia Screening Programme, which in many cases enables young adults to send in their swabs via the post. However, please beware of commercial testing kits which give women an instant 'on-the-spot' result – these are not to be relied on.

NAATs are now the gold-standard test for the detection of chlamydial infection, and are widely available. Vaginal self swabs have been found to be more accurate than first-catch urine samples in females as they pick up a higher bacterial load, and such swabbing has become the standard investigation for the National Chlamydia Screening Programme. Swabs can be taken by a clinician during examination, or the woman can swab herself safe with the knowledge that vaginal self-swabbing has been found to be as sensitive as cervical swabbing in detecting chlamydial infection.

In the case of self-swabbing, the woman should be instructed to wipe her vulva with tissue paper, then part the labia. She should then pass the swab high into the vagina and rub it several times against the vaginal walls. She then resheathes the swab, replaces it into its plastic cover and into the testing bag. She should wash her hands, seal the bag, and hand the specimen in (or post it as instructed). In areas of high gonorrhoea prevalence, NAAT swabs may be tested for gonorrhoea as well as chlamydia (check with your local laboratory to see whether this is the case or not).

If the result of the NAAT swab is positive for chlamydia or gonorrhoea, antibiotic sensitivities cannot be ascertained by a NAAT test. It is, therefore, important for GPs to be up to date with local protocols, which can change frequently. At the time of writing, Azithromycin 1g stat is the standard treatment for chlamydia, and cefixime 400mg stat is the standard treatment for gonorrhoea.

GOOD PRACTICE POINT 1.9

- Make sure that you check with your local microbiology laboratory or sexual health clinic what the current antibiotic protocols are for the treatment of chlamydia and gonorrhoea before prescribing. Looking at the BNF alone is not acceptable.

Charcoal swabs

Black charcoal microbiology swabs have numerous functions, and are used by doctors and nurses to swab almost anywhere on the body that looks infected. They are important in the area of women's health as they can be used to swab the high vagina to test for thrush, bacterial vaginosis, gonorrhoea, trichomonas and group B streptococcus. The results from a charcoal swab usually come with antibiotic sensitivities for any bacterial organisms found. If the swab reports the presence of clue cells, this can be interpreted as the presence of bacterial vaginosis if the woman is symptomatic for this (fishy smelling discharge), but can be ignored otherwise as it is often a result of no significance. All women who have tested positive for gonorrhoea on NAAT testing should have a charcoal swab done: (i) to confirm the result; (ii) to check treatment given is appropriate by determining the antibiotic sensitivity of the organism; and (iii) as a public health measure to enable local protocols to be changed as required. It should be noted that a high vaginal charcoal swab will not test reliably for gonorrhoea; to be sure of the result, a specimen must be collected from the cervix, and ideally from the urethra as well. In addition, in circumstances where the woman has practiced anal or oral sex, charcoal swabs should be taken from the rectum and throat as appropriate.

Viral swabs

Viral swabs should only be used on women with an open genital ulcer. If there is no ulceration seen, the result will come back as negative. The lid of the ulcer should be gently lifted off with a needle if it has crusted over, then the swab must be rubbed quite firmly on the base of the ulcer in order to have a fair chance of harvesting any viral organisms present. It is useful if an outbreak of herpes can be confirmed by viral swabbing in this way, not only to be sure of the diagnosis, but also the report will indicate whether the infection is due to herpes simplex type I or II, which have different prognoses (see Module 7).

GOOD PRACTICE POINT 1.10

- Know what swabs should be taken for each condition.

Cervical cytology

Liquid-based cytology is now the method used in the cervical screening programme. It acts to harvest cells from the transformation zone of the uterine cervix for examination under a light microscope. It is a slightly invasive test, and most women dislike having it done. It is, therefore, important that the woman is made to feel at ease, and that her initial apprehension is alleviated. The cervix is visualised with the use of a disposable Cusco speculum (it is important that no lubricant is used to insert this as lubricant alters the cytology results). If there is a mucus plug in the cervical os, this should be gently removed with a clean swab. The tip of a cytology brush is then placed into the cervical os, and the brush swept a full 360°, 5–8 times. The head of the brush is then removed from the cervix and dipped several times in a collection pot which is then sent to a laboratory for analysis. In some areas, the head of the cytology brush is snapped off and left in the collection pot. The pot must be labelled correctly otherwise the laboratory staff will reject the sample. The woman should be told that results can take up to 8 weeks to come through, and not to worry should that be the case. If you are concerned that the woman has a serious condition that needs attention (such as post-menopausal bleeding), then she should be referred urgently to the gynaecology clinic without waiting for the cervical cytology results.

All healthcare professionals who take cervical cytology need to have regular updates, and must register with their PCT as a cytology sample taker. It is good practice to audit your own results, checking each result that comes back, and noting down the number of 'inadequate' results you get compared to colleagues.

IMAGING INVESTIGATIONS

Ultrasound scans

Ultrasound scans are cheap, safe, and usually easily accessible. Many women feel quite re-assured by having one done, more so than simply being examined. Ultrasound investigations are a useful tool for the worried patient as they produce no harmful radiation. An ultrasound scanner works on a similar principle to the radar of submarines, producing real-time images of otherwise unseen organs by the use of reflected sound waves. Sound waves are directed into the body via a probe, organs absorb some of the waves, and the remaining waves are reflected back to the probe as an echo. A computer analyses the pattern of these echoes, and produces a visual image on a monitor that can be seen by the ultrasonographer. As the sound waves are high above the human hearing range, we hear nothing.

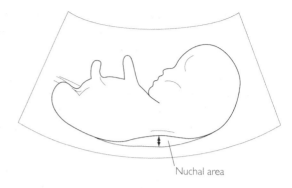

Nuchal area

The transvaginal probe is the preferred method used to visualise the pelvic organs of a female. The transabdominal probe is only used to visualise the

Figure 1.7 Illustration of ultrasound scan at 12 weeks.

pelvis if the woman is a virgin, otherwise unable to tolerate transvaginal scanning (for example, vaginitis), or transvaginal scanning is unavailable which may be the case as it requires an ultrasonographer with specialist training. The transabdominal probe has the advantage that it can also be used to visualise organs of the abdomen as well as pelvis, and it is of course the probe used for men and children.

An ultrasound scan is the investigation of choice in the following circumstances:

- To assess IUD placement (in the case of lost threads).

- To assess and monitor the fetus during pregnancy (Fig. 1.7). The transvaginal probe is preferred for first trimester scanning; the abdominal probe for second and third trimester scanning.

- To diagnose and monitor ectopic pregnancy.

- To measure the thickness and regularity of the endometrium in post-menopausal bleeding.

- To determine the location and measure the size of uterine fibroids.

- To assess any ovarian pathology such as cysts.

- To assess pelvic mass.

- To monitor fertility treatment. Ultrasound scanning is used to determine the number and quality of follicles that are developing in the ovary during superovulation therapy and egg harvesting.

- To assess the quality and size of breast lumps, particularly those in young women.

- To locate lost contraceptive implants. This requires a clinician who has been specially trained in the technique.

Doppler ultrasound

Doppler ultrasound scanning is used as a way of assessing blood flow. It uses reflected sound waves specifically to evaluate blood as it flows through a vessel. It is a particularly useful technique in pregnancy as it allows the blood flow between the fetus and placenta to be visualised. By using repeated Doppler ultrasound scanning, placental insufficiency can be closely monitored. This helps provide obstetricians with the information they need to decide when best to deliver a compromised fetus.

Doppler ultrasound scanning is also useful in the assessment of the angiogenesis (growth of new blood vessels) which occurs in many cancers, and in assessing the blood supply of fibroids prior to myomectomy.

Radiography

To the annoyance of radiologists, most people inaccurately refer to radiographs as X-rays. A radiograph is an image produced on a photograph film caused by X-rays (a type of electromagnetic radiation wave) hitting it. The X-rays are directed at the photographic film and the part of the person being X-rayed (e.g. the pelvis) is put between the film and the X-ray machine. The tissues that lie in the path of the X-ray beam absorb the X-ray differently, and this is captured in the image. The impact on society of this technique has been immense.

Radiographs are contra-indicated during pregnancy; if there is any chance of pregnancy, most radiographers will refuse to take a radiograph without a lot of persuasion, and the covering of the woman's abdomen and pelvis with a lead jacket. This is because it is known that radiation can be harmful to a developing fetus.

In the realm of obstetrics and gynaecology, abdominal radiographs are only really useful to locate an intra-uterine device that has perforated through the uterine wall, or, occasionally, to assess a foreign body such as glass in the vagina; glass shows up well on X-ray but is not so easily seen on inspection.

Mammography

Mammography is a radiograph (taken with X-rays) of the breast. It is effective in identifying breast lumps in women before they have become large enough to be found by breast examination. As the prognosis of breast cancer is so much better the earlier the cancer is found, and because breast cancer is such a common and devastating disease, in the UK all women are invited to have mammograms regularly between the ages of 50–65 years as part of the breast cancer screening programme. Mammography is only really suitable for women over the age of 40 years. This is because prior to this age the breast tissue, under the influence of oestrogen, is too dense to distinguish lumps from normal tissue.

Women should be advised that having a mammogram can be slightly uncomfortable as each breast must be held quite tightly between two plates. Deodorant, talcum powder and body lotion can all show up as calcium spots, so women should not apply this on the day of the investigation.

GOOD PRACTICE POINT 1.11

- Women are still recommended to examine their own breasts on a regular basis, but this advice is controversial.

Despite the inconvenience, most women look forward to mammography due to the great re-assurance it can provide if the result is negative, and the early treatment options available if the result is positive. All women with a positive result are automatically referred on to a breast surgeon for examination and biopsy. There is a high rate of false positive mammography results, which means that up to a third of women referred onto a surgeon turn out to be all clear. Unfortunately, mammography has a false negative rate of at least 10%, which means that one in ten breast cancers is missed.

Computed tomography (CT) scans

Computed tomography is referred to as CT scanning in the UK, CAT scanning in the USA, and even as 'the donut' to some patients. It makes use of serial X-rays and advanced computer technology to generate a multi-layered image that can be used to build a three-dimensional picture. As with plain radiographs, CT scans are contra-indicated in pregnancy due to the adverse effects of radiation on the fetus.

In the field of obstetrics and gynaecology, CT scans are usually reserved for the assessment of pelvic cancers, their lymph node involvement and metastases.

Magnetic resonance imaging (MRI) scans

Magnetic resonance imaging is a very expensive and limited resource. It has the great advantage of being radiation free, but involves the patient lying in a long tube which many find claustrophobic, for up to an hour. The scanner is quite noisy, so patients are given ear plugs to wear during the scan. MRI is not appropriate for women with pacemakers or prosthetic joints, but an IUD is allowable (it can slip during MRI scanning if newly inserted, but this is unusual).

MRI, as its name suggests, makes use of magnetism. Intermittent radio waves, up to 30,000 times stronger than the magnetic field of the earth, are beamed through the patient. Due to the charged nature of all particles and atoms, such strong magnetism forces each atom of the body to align. When the magnetism is turned off, the aligned atoms revert to their original random distribution, emitting radio waves of their own as they do so. The scanner picks up these signals and a computer turns them into a picture.

MRI has a number of specialist roles. In particular, it is the gold standard investigation in the monitoring of endometrial carcinoma, and, in particular, any myometrial invasion by the same.

Hysteroscopy

Hysteroscopy is the name given to the procedure used to have a direct look at the inside of the uterus. The hysteroscope is a small, flexible, fibre-optic camera that is navigated by a skilled gynaecologist through the cervix into the uterus. Sometimes, slight dilatation of the cervix is required to allow the hysteroscope to pass. Saline or carbon dioxide is gently introduced into the uterine cavity, which stretches the usually opposed uterine walls and allows viewing of the cavity. The hysteroscope produces real-time pictures of the uterine cavity which are interpreted by computer and sent digitally to a monitor for viewing. Hysteroscopy can be performed under general or local anaesthesia.

Hysteroscopy is useful when there is diagnostic uncertainty, such as unexplained pelvic pain or unexplained inter-menstrual bleeding. Hysteroscopy is also useful to investigate persistent menorrhagia, and post-menopausal bleeding. Hysteroscopy can visualise a uterine malformation. If an abnormality is found, an operative hysteroscope is the invaluable tool that comes into play; it has a channel incorporated within its structure to allow the passage of specialised instruments. Using an operative hysteroscope, the gynaecologist is able to take an endometrial biopsy, excise an endometrial polyp or submucosal fibroid, or perform other specialised surgery.

LEGAL AND ETHICAL ISSUES

LEGAL STATUS OF THE UNBORN CHILD

In the UK, a fetus has no legal rights; the life of the mother is always paramount. The mother has the freedom to refuse treatment that may potentially save the life of the fetus, including emergency caesarean section. Once a baby has been delivered, he or she has the full rights of any human being, and the mother is not allowed to refuse treatment for her child.

At any time during the pregnancy, right up to the time of delivery, feticide is legal in the UK if there is a known significant fetal abnormality. However, once the baby has been born, even if the baby was born pre-maturely and has severe disability, infanticide is illegal. This is an ethical contradiction, and a matter of considerable public and parliamentary debate. A number of prominent ethicists, in particular Peter Singer, have debated this at length.

Fetal abnormalities that allow the mother to proceed to a late termination of pregnancy (up to term) must be 'of a substantial risk that if the child were born it would suffer from such physical or mental abnormalities as to be seriously handicapped'. Antenatal recognition of fetal malformations relies on accurate detection from screening programmes using either maternal serum screening, routine ultrasound scanning, or a combination of both. Most fetal abnormalities can be recognised at 12 weeks' gestation or soon afterwards using a variety of methods (see Module 3) but there are some conditions in which malformations only become clear after 24 weeks of gestation. Examples of such are hypoplastic left heart syndrome and cerebral ventriculomegaly.

It is recognised by obstetricians that it is often not possible to predict the seriousness of outcome of a fetal abnormality, either in terms of the long-term physical, intellectual or social disability on the child, or the knock on effects to the family. The RCOG believes that the interpretation of 'serious abnormality' should be based upon individual discussion between the parents and the doctor. There are no strict guidelines on this and no list of conditions that are accepted as 'serious enough' to allow late abortion. For this reason, many conditions sit on the fence, causing decision making, in some cases, to be excruciatingly painful. One such controversial example of this includes sickle cell anaemia; a good quality and productive life can be lead by some individuals, but recurrent painful crises, suffering and disability are endured by others. Cystic fibrosis is another common disease over which terminating a pregnancy is vigorously debated.

MEDICAL CONFIDENTIALITY

Confidentiality is central to trust between doctors and patients. Without assurances about confidentiality, patients can become reluctant to provide doctors with the information they need in order to provide good care. For this reason, patient data should be anonymised where unidentifiable data will serve the purpose, healthcare professionals should never discuss patient's problems in any place where there is a possibility that they can be overheard, and patient records should never be left where they can be seen by others, either on paper or screen. All reasonable steps should be taken to ensure that consultations are private.

Confidentiality for women under 16 years of age is a very sensitive issue. There is an intrinsic struggle between wanting to treat these women with respect and provide confidentiality, while at the same time safeguarding them against harm. It is essential that all healthcare providers who care for young women are adequately trained and prepared in order that they are able to deal appropriately, safely and sensitively with any situations that arise.

You should usually share information about sexual activity involving children under 13 years, as these are considered in law to be unable to consent. You should discuss a decision not to disclose with a named or designated doctor for child protection, and record your decision with the reasons for it.

Gillick/Fraser competence

Mrs Gillick, a mother of 10 children (five girls and five boys), brought a declaration before the House of Lords in 1985 that prescribing contraception to under 16-year-old girls was illegal because the doctor would commit an offence of encouraging sex with a minor, and that it would be treatment without consent from the parent. The issue before the House of Lords was whether a young lady had the capacity to give consent for herself, without involving a parent, and it was agreed that they could as long as they understood the decision they were making.

In 1989, Lord Fraser honed the law in specific relation to prescribing contraceptives to under 16-year-old girls without the knowledge of their parents. It was decided that it is lawful for doctors to provide contraceptive advice and treatment without parental consent providing certain criteria are met. These criteria are:

- The young lady understands the professional's advice.
- The young lady cannot be persuaded to inform their parents, and does not want the doctor to inform the parents.
- The young lady is very likely to begin, or to continue having, sexual intercourse with or without contraceptive treatment.
- Unless the young lady receives contraceptive treatment, their physical or mental health, or both, are likely to suffer.
- The young lady's best interests require them to receive contraceptive advice or treatment with or without parental consent.

These criteria specifically refer to contraception but the principles are also applied to abortion and, although the judgement in the House of Lords referred specifically to doctors, it is considered to apply to other health professionals as well, such as nurses.

GOOD PRACTICE POINT 1.12

- Know what your practice policy is on seeing unaccompanied under 16-year-old girls.

Safeguarding

A confidential sexual health service is essential for the welfare of children and young people. Concern about confidentiality is the biggest deterrent to young people asking for sexual health advice. That, in turn, presents dangers to young people's own health and to that of the community, particularly other young people.

You may not be able to judge whether a relationship is abusive without knowing the identity of a young person's sexual partner, which the young person might not want to reveal. If you are concerned that a relationship is abusive, you should carefully balance the benefits of knowing a sexual partner's identity against the potential loss of trust in asking for or sharing such information.

The GMC have extensive advice regarding the safeguarding of children and young people. It is recommended that all clinicians who deal with this potentially vulnerable patient group become familiar with the GMC website and keep themselves up-to-date with current guidance.

USEFUL WEBSITE

- Full GMC guidance on the safeguarding of children and young people can be found at: <www.gmc-uk.org/guidance/ethical_guidance/children_guidance/64_69_sexual_activity.asp>

Children below the age of 13 years

The GP should usually share information about sexual activity involving any child under the age of 13 years, who are considered in law to be unable to consent. Any decision not to disclose information should be discussed with the local designated doctor for child protection and the decision recorded in the medical notes, along with the reasons for the same.

Harmful sexual activity

The GP can disclose relevant information when this is in the public interest. If a child or young person is involved in abusive or seriously harmful sexual activity, you must protect them by sharing relevant information with the appropriate people or agencies, such as the police or social services, quickly and professionally. The GP should consider each case on its merits and take into account the young person's behaviour, living circumstances, maturity, serious learning disabilities, and any other factors that might make them particularly vulnerable.

Knowledge about harmful sexual activity involving a young person that should usually be shared is that which involves the following:

- A young person too immature to understand or consent.
- Big differences in age, maturity or power between sexual partners.
- A young person's sexual partner having a position of trust, such as a foster carer, teacher, or doctor.
- Force or the threat of force, emotional or psychological pressure, bribery or payment, either to engage in sexual activity or to keep it secret.
- Drugs or alcohol used to influence a young person to engage in sexual activity when they otherwise would not.
- A person known to the police or child protection agencies as having had abusive relationships with children or young people who is continuing to do so.

MEDICAL CERTIFICATION

Prescription exemption

Mother's are currently entitled to free prescriptions throughout the pregnancy, and for 12 months after delivery. The pregnant lady needs to complete Form FW8 in order to claim this, the form is available from GPs or midwives.

MATERNITY PAY AND BENEFITS

It is important that before giving advice you look at the Government website for up-to-date information on benefits, as the eligibility criteria and amounts paid change frequently.

Alternatively, women can be referred directly to their local Citizens Advice Bureau for up-to-date information on benefits. Midwives are also an invaluable source of information and expertise in this area.

USEFUL WEBSITES

- <www.direct.gov.uk/en/MoneyTaxAndBenefits/BenefitsTaxCreditsAndOtherSupport/ Expectingorbringingupchildren>

<www.everychildmatters.gov.uk>

Statutory maternity pay

Below are listed a number of general points of information regarding statutory maternity pay (SMP):

- SMP is paid by the employer (so the unemployed do not get it, nor do the self-employed).
- If a woman holds more than one permanent job, she may be able to get SMP from each employer.
- Receiving SMP does not mean the mother has to return to work for that employer afterwards.
- Remember that income tax and national insurance must be paid on it.

Maternity allowance

Below are listed a number of general points of information regarding maternity allowance (MA):

- MA is for those who are employed, but not eligible for SMP; this includes those women who have not been in their current job long enough to qualify for SMP, women who changed jobs during pregnancy, and women who did not earn enough to qualify for SMP.
- MA is also for the self-employed.
- MA is not paid by the employer, it is paid directly by the Government's Department of Work and Pensions.

Maternity leave

Below are listed a number of points of information regarding maternity leave:

- All women must take at least 2 weeks leave following birth, those who work in factories must take at least 4 weeks.
- Apart from that, women can choose when to start their maternity leave and how long they want to take. All pregnant employees are currently entitled to take up to one year of maternity leave, regardless of length of service with the employer.
- The first 26 weeks taken are known as 'Ordinary Maternity Leave'. During this time, the woman should receive all of her contractual benefits.
- The second 26 weeks taken are known as 'Additional Maternity Leave', and must directly follow Ordinary Maternity Leave. Benefits will depend on the employment contract, and may be unpaid in many cases.

Statutory paternity pay

Statutory paternity pay (SPP) is paid by employers for up to 2 consecutive weeks after the birth of a child to men whose partner gives birth to, or adopts, an infant. SPP is currently available to:

- The baby's biological father.

- The mother's partner.
- The man responsible for the baby's upbringing.
- A female partner in a same sex couple.

Paternity leave

For those who do not qualify for SPP, such as those who have not been in their current job long enough, negotiation needs to take place directly with the employer to arrange unpaid leave, or paid annual leave. For the self-employed, own arrangements will need to be made. There is currently no equivalent of maternity allowance for men.

Parental leave

All mothers in the UK currently have the right to take up to 13 weeks unpaid time off work to look after a child, up until the child's fifth birthday (or 18th birthday for disabled children). This is known as 'parental leave'.

Module 2: Basic surgical skills

You will be expected to demonstrate an understanding of commonly performed obstetric and gynaecological surgical procedures including their complications.

You will need to be aware of commonly encountered infections, including an understanding of the principles of infection control.

You will be expected to interpret pre-operative investigations and be aware of the principles involved in appropriate pre-operative and postoperative care.

You will be expected to understand the legal issues surrounding consent in all clinical situations including termination of pregnancy.

THE WOMAN PRESENTING TO THE GYNAECOLOGIST

This chapter discusses a number of common surgical techniques, and aims to familiarise the reader with the routine work of a gynaecologist. The information is presented at a level suitable for a gynaecology specialist trainee, and provides insight for GPs who have not done a gynaecology job. This chapter is not intended to teach doctors how to operate, but rather to understand surgical procedures so that accurate information can be given to patients, both before and after surgical treatment.

PRE-OPERATIVE CARE

PRE-OPERATIVE INVESTIGATIONS

Pre-admission clinic is becoming increasingly a nurse-led service. Protocols are strictly followed to ensure that patient safety is maintained. Blood pressure should be within a normal range. Almost all pre-anaesthetic admissions have a full blood count done, especially in gynaecology where women are often anaemic. Where blood loss is envisaged, a blood sample is taken for 'group-and-save' in case a blood transfusion becomes necessary. A haemoglobinopathy screen is done if appropriate, and, if necessary, renal and liver function testing is performed.

CONSENT

Consent can be defined as an agreement by a patient to receive treatment, undergo a procedure or participate in research. The GMC insists that every doctor must be satisfied that they have consent or other valid authority before undertaking any examination or investigation, providing treatment or involving patients in teaching or research. For consent to be valid:

- The patient must be assessed as having the capacity to consent.

- The patient must be provided with sufficient information, in a way that they can understand, in order to make an informed choice. This involves explaining the risks and benefits of the treatment, and discussing the alternatives.

The patient must have given the consent freely and without coercion. Pressurising the patient into consenting to treatment invalidates the consent. To ensure that consent is freely given, patients should, where possible, be given time to consider their options before making their decision. For this reason, consent is best obtained in an out-patient clinic and not on the ward on the day of admission. Coercion by friends or relatives to have a procedure also invalidates consent. This is of particular concern for consent to termination of pregnancy, where the influence of others can be considerable.

USEFUL WEBSITE

- <http://www.gmc-uk.org/guidance/ethical_guidance/consent_guidance/expressions_of_consent.asp>

There are different types of consent

Implied consent

Implied consent is when consent is assumed by interpreting the unspoken actions of a patient. An example of this is a patient who stretches out her arm towards a nurse when asked if blood pressure can be taken.

Verbal consent

Verbal consent when a patient vocalises their agreement to a procedure. This is usual practice prior to performing an examination of the genitalia, or inserting a contraceptive implant.

Written consent

Written consent involves the patient signing on a consent form as a demonstration of their agreement to a procedure. There are very few occasions where the law specifically requires written consent; one example is when treatment involves the storage and use of gametes and embryos in fertility treatment. Nevertheless, most hospitals require consent forms to be completed prior to a patient undergoing surgery. Generally speaking, verbal consent is just as valid as written consent. Consent is a process resulting in an agreement, not a signature on a form. Therefore, it is important to realise that completed consent forms provide some evidence that consent was obtained, but little beyond that. Consent forms do not in themselves constitute proof that the consent was valid.

Presumed consent

Presumed consent is when a doctor or nurse acts in an emergency situation for the patient's best interest, presuming that is what they would want. Such is the case in the event of an accident, or following a cardiac arrest. During such emergencies, it is impossible to gain informed consent, as the patient is either too confused, too fatigued, or unconscious. In such situations, the healthcare team must act in the patient's best interest. If there is a known advanced directive, this must be taken into account so that there is adherence to the patient's wishes.

Consent by proxy

In the UK, the Mental Capacity Act, 2005 (implemented in 2007) allows consent to be given by proxy. This is a change in the law, and aligns English law with Scottish law. This change means that, if an adult is incapacitated, consent can be given on their behalf by a named proxy. This is usually a family member, the next of kin or a carer who is nominated to have Lasting Power of Attorney for the patient's health issues. In the absence of a proxy decision-maker, either because none exists or because the proxy cannot be reached, the doctor should act in the patient's best interest. In Scotland, another person can give consent on behalf of an incapacitated adult.

Consent in the young
For consent from young people see Module 7.

GOOD PRACTICE POINT 2.1

- Remember to record consent for all procedures in the medical notes.

PERI-OPERATIVE CARE

INFECTION CONTROL

Postoperative wound infections are common, and are a risk of any surgery. Wound infection delays recovery, increases length of stay in hospital, causes pain and discomfort to the patient, and may result in the formation of a sub-optimal scar. In severe cases, postoperative infection can lead to systemic infection, septicaemia, and death. The prevention of postoperative infection is, therefore, of great importance.

Certain population groups are at a higher risk of postoperative infection than others. Recognising this increased susceptibility is important as often extra steps can be taken to prevent infection occurring in these women. Risk factors can be classified for convenience of the memory as relating to the patient, the procedure, the surgical team, the equipment, and the environment.

The patient
Extremes of age increase susceptibility to infection; therefore, the very young and the very old are at high risk. Concurrent disease, such as diabetes, immunosuppression or cancer also increases the likelihood of contracting infection.

The procedure
Certain procedures carry a higher risk of infection than others. Long operating times generally indicate a high risk. Instrumentation or incision into infected tissue (e.g. operating on an ectopic pregnancy in the presence of active pelvic inflammatory disease) or incision of the bowel carries a high risk of postoperative infection than other procedures.

The surgical team
It has been shown that poor surgical technique and procedures, carried out by surgeons with insufficient training, results in higher rates of postoperative infection. Poor attention to hygiene in particular is a direct cause of postoperative infection. Simple washing with soaps or detergents is, therefore, the most important component of infection control. Staff should wash their hands on arrival at work, and before departure. Staff should also wash their hands before and after examining a patient.

Poor attention to hygiene directly results in higher rates of infection. This includes inappropriate use of theatre clothing and insufficient time spent washing hands.

During all invasive procedures, it is mandatory that gloves are worn by staff. Non-sterile gloves can be worn on both hands for pelvic examination and speculum examination. Sterile gloves should be worn during any surgical procedure, including colposcopy, and when examining a woman in labour.

The equipment
All instruments used in community clinics and general practice should be single-use only and all instruments must be

disposed of safely. This involves sharps being deposited in a sharps bin, and all instruments that have been in contact with bodily fluids being deposited in special contamination bins for incineration. This includes latex gloves, plastic aprons, and vaginal speculums.

Inadequate sterilisation of equipment or re-use of equipment can lead to high postoperative infection rates. Inappropriate dressings can render a wound more susceptible to infection.

Wound drains are a port of entry for bacteria, causing increased infection rates so should only be used when absolutely necessary, and certainly not as an alternative to good haemostasis during the procedure.

The environment

It is compulsory that every hospital and clinic in the UK has robust procedures in place to ensure that infection is not transmitted between patients, and between staff and patients. There should be an infection control policy in every clinical centre that has been designed and implemented by an infection control team. Such a team usually consists of a consultant microbiologist, specialist nurses and, possibly, a junior doctor.

Inadequate operating theatre ventilation, simultaneous operations in the same room, and unrestricted movement of staff all act to increase infection rates. This is because turbulent airflow increases the quantity of air-borne bacteria such as *Staphylococcus aureus* and β-haemolytic streptococci. For this reason, staff with a boil, septic skin lesion, or eczema colonised with methicillin-resistant *S. aureus* (MRSA) should not be allowed into the operating theatre. Theatre gowns should not be worn outside the operating department.

Prolonged pre- or postoperative stays in hospital increase infection rates, even when known carriers of infectious disease are isolated.

DISINFECTANTS

Disinfectants are chemicals that kill or inhibit microbes.

Chlorhexidine is active against bacteria, especially Staphylococcus spp. (including MRSA).

Alcohol acts rapidly against bacteria and viruses, and enhances the disinfecting power of antiseptics such as chlorhexidine. Alcohol is used with chlorhexidine in hand washes such as Hibiscrub, the first-line choice for disinfection of hands. Alcohol gel can be used to cleanse the hands as long as there is no visible dirt on them. Hands should only be cleansed using an alcohol gel three times before washing with water and detergent.

Iodine-based compounds are most active against bacteria, but are relatively slow acting. Iodine-based washes can be used for disinfection of the patient's skin before performing surgery.

Hypochlorite compounds, such as bleach, are most active against viruses. Hypochlorite is used to disinfect surfaces and floors. It is responsible for the familiar smell of swimming pools.

Phenolic disinfectants are highly active against bacteria, and are used to disinfect contaminated surfaces. They are also found in weaker formulation antiseptics such as Dettol, and in mouthwashes.

Disinfecting the patient before treatment

- Prior to venepuncture or arteropuncture, the skin of the patient should be wiped with an alcohol pre-injection swab.

- Prior to skin incision in a patient undergoing surgery, the skin should be cleaned thoroughly using a skin disinfectant such as 20% chlorhexidine in surfactant solution, or 10% povidone–iodine solution. Disinfectants with greater than 40% alcohol content should be avoided if diathermy is going to be used, as severe burns can result. The antiseptic should be applied with friction for 3–4 minutes, and must be allowed to dry before operating.

- The cervix of a patient undergoing colposcopy should be cleaned using normal saline.

- The cervix of a patient undergoing hysteroscopy, termination of pregnancy or removal of retained products of conception should be cleaned using antiseptic wash or normal saline.

STERILISATION

Sterilisation kills all infectious organisms and can be achieved by a number of methods. Autoclaving involves heating surgical instruments with superheated pressurised steam. Gamma-irradiation is used during manufacture of perishable materials such as plastic cannulae, syringes, and uterine sounds.

Soaking equipment in formaldehyde can sterilise instruments if they are adequately cleaned first. This method is popular in some underdeveloped countries, but is not used in the UK, where more fastidious techniques are preferred.

SURGICAL INSTRUMENTS

Below are diagrams of some common surgical instruments used by gynaecologists that you should become familiar with. Instruments are generally made of high-grade surgical steel which can be autoclaved for repeat use, or prepared for single-use only.

The uterine sound (Fig. 2.1) is inserted gently through the cervical os in order to measure the length of the uterine cavity.

Volsellum forceps (Fig. 2.2) are toothed forceps used to grip the cervix. By so doing, the uterus is stabilised for instrumentation. Volsellum forceps may be straight or curved. They may also be referred to as Tenaculum, or Allis forceps.

Vaginal specula include the Cusco speculum (Fig. 2.3) and Sims speculum (Fig. 2.4).

Scissors (Fig. 2.5) are all single-use only. There are many uses for scissors, including the trimming of IUD threads, loosening of adhesions, debridement of wounds, performing episiotomy, and cutting of the umbilical cord.

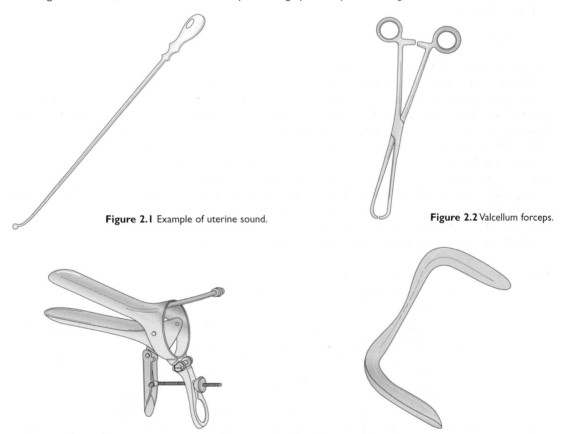

Figure 2.1 Example of uterine sound.

Figure 2.2 Valcellum forceps.

Figure 2.3 Cusco speculum.

Figure 2.4 Sims speculum.

Cervical dilators (Fig. 2.6) come in sizes known as Hegar. A Hegar 3 cervical dilator is the smallest size in general usage. It should fit easily through the cervical os, even that of a nulliparous woman. A cervical dilator sized Hegar 4 is slightly larger. A copper IUD is the size of Hagar 4. A cervical dilator sized Hegar 5 is larger still, but will still often fit easily through the cervical os of a parous woman, although it can bit a bit more difficult a nulliparous woman, or a woman with cervical stenosis. The Mirena coil is the size of Hagar 5. Dilators sized Hegar 6 and 7 are used for insertion of a hysteroscope. Dilators sized Hegar 8, 9 and 10 are used for late terminations of pregnancy and evacuation of retained products of conception (ERPC). Dilating the cervix to such a size is difficult, and the cervix should be primed with the insertion of vaginal misoprostal 4 hours before the procedure.

Curettes (Fig. 2.7) come in different shapes and sizes. They are used for curettage of the uterine cavity, what some women refer to as 'the scrape'.

POSTOPERATIVE CARE

Ideally, all patients should be seen by their operating surgeon within the 24 hours following their procedure. Follow-up should be arranged with the patient whenever required, whether that be with the surgeon in an out-patient clinic, with their GP, or with a specialist nurse. Contraception should be in place if indicated, or a clear plan in place to start such. Advice should be given to all women as to whom they should consult and where they can receive help, should they need advice or develop a problem. All women should be made aware of known complications of their procedure, and how they should manage them. Prophylactic antibiotics and analgesics may be prescribed, depending on the procedure and the clinical judgement of the doctor or nurse practitioner.

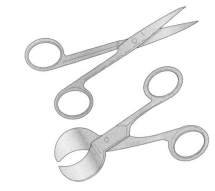

Figure 2.5 Examples of scissors.

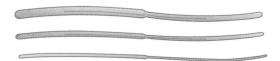

Figure 2.6 Cervical dilators.

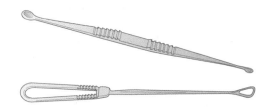

Figure 2.7 Curettes.

ADHESIONS

Adhesions are fibrous bands that form between tissues and internal organs. In the realm of women's health, adhesions are a known complication of any surgery to the pelvis and of many gynaecological conditions, including caesarean section, pelvic inflammatory disease and endometriosis. Adhesions are a result of normal wound healing; during surgery, inflammatory cells from the injured tissue (macrophages and T-lymphocytes) release histamine, cytokines and growth factors as an immediate inflammatory response, while fibroblasts from the muscle release fibrin. Together, these factors form of a tough extracellular matrix as part of the normal healing process, the matrix forming a glue that seals the injury. However, the matrix, as well as joining the incised tissues back together, often also results in joining tissues together that should be separate. Such abnormal fibrous connections are what are known as adhesions.

Adhesions may be asymptomatic and, if so, require no treatment. However, adhesions can fix organs which are usually mobile (such as the uterus) to the pelvis or to the surgical incision site. This can result in chronic pelvic pain, and dyspareunia which can be very difficult to manage. Adhesions can also be a cause of subfertility. Surgery to release the adhesions often results only in more adhesions being formed, but can give temporary relief.

Surgeons and pharmaceutical companies have developed a number of methods to try to minimise postoperative adhesion formation.

SURGICAL TREATMENTS FOR HEAVY MENSTRUAL BLEEDING

ENDOMETRIAL ABLATION

Endometrial ablation is a technique used to improve the problem of heavy menstrual bleeding when medical treatments and the intra-uterine system have failed to help symptoms adequately. Endometrial ablation employs a number of techniques to ablate (remove) the full depth of the endometrium. It can be performed under general or local anaesthesia. The aim of treatment is to stop menstrual periods or make them considerably lighter. Endometrial ablation is a very successful procedure, particularly in women who are over 40 years old, who may otherwise have considered a hysterectomy. Up to 90% of women will have greatly reduced menstrual bleeds after treatment, with up to half becoming amenorrhoeic. This can be a great relief for women who may have been suffering from menorrhagia for many years.

Preparation for treatment

Prior to the procedure, the woman is often provided with 4–6 weeks of oral hormone therapy which acts to suppress endometrial growth. The most common drug used for this is a GnRH analogue such as Zoladex 3.6 mg subcutaneous injection, 1 month before treatment. Endometrial suppression in this way has been shown to improve treatment outcome significantly.

Postoperative care

By removing the full depth of the endometrium, permanent infertility will be caused in most women after treatment. Therefore, endometrial ablation is not an appropriate treatment for women who have not yet completed their family. However, endometrial ablation is not a contraceptive method, and ectopic pregnancies in particular are a real possibility following treatment. Women who have undergone endometrial ablation therapy should, therefore, be strongly advised to take up use of a reliable effective contraceptive method. Sterilisation is offered by some centres at the same time as the endometrial treatment.

MYOMECTOMY

Myomectomy is the name given to the surgical procedure of removing fibroids from the uterus. This operation is reserved for women with troublesome fibroids who do not want a hysterectomy. It is performed under general or spinal anaesthesia. Depending on the location and size of the fibroids, myomectomy may be carried out hysteroscopically, laparoscopically or via laparotomy.

Myomectomy can result in extensive blood loss and it is important that the patient appreciates this before agreeing to the operation. Some units use intra-operative cell salvage to recycle the patient's own blood, but many women will need a transfusion of donated blood on top of the salvaged blood. It is also important that she understands that, by retaining her uterus, she may grow new fibroids in the future.

An alternative is fibroid embolisation, which is performed by a specialist interventional radiographer, under sedation. Microspheres are injected into the uterine artery, with the aim of reducing blood flow to the fibroid and causing it to shrink. Complications include infection, emboli in other organs, ovarian damage, pain and foul vaginal odour as necrotic tissue is expelled. However, fibroid embolisation may give a faster recovery time than open myomectomy, and in expert hands can be very satisfactory.

HYSTERECTOMY

Hysterectomy is the term given to the surgical procedure of removing the uterus. Indications for a hysterectomy include:

- Severe menorrhagia when other treatments have failed.
- Severe endometriosis or adenomyosis where other treatments have failed.
- Uterine, ovarian or cervical cancer.

- As an emergency, life-saving procedure in certain post-partum situations, e.g. placenta accreta or severe post-partum haemorrhage.

- As a prophylactic treatment along with oophorectomy and salpingectomy for those with a strong family history of reproductive system cancers.

- Occasionally, as part of gender re-assignment surgery, along with oophorectomy and salpingectomy, before the construction of male genitalia.

Total hysterectomy

Total hysterectomy, as its name suggests, involves the removal of the whole uterus from the pelvis. This includes the uterine body, uterine fundus and the complete cervix. Women who have undergone a total hysterectomy should be removed from the cervical screening programme unless the hysterectomy was performed as a treatment for cervical cancer; in those cases, annual vault smears may be advised.

Subtotal hysterectomy

Subtotal hysterectomy involves removal of the uterine body and fundus only, leaving the cervical stump in position. Women who have undergone subtotal hysterectomy should remain in the cervical screening programme as normal, as they have the same risk as any other woman of developing cervical neoplasia. Patients must be warned about this before undergoing the operation. Subtotal hysterectomy has the benefits of a quicker, less complex operation with, usually, fewer postoperative complications, and less disruption to bladder and sexual function.

GOOD PRACTICE POINT 2.2

- Make sure you understand the difference between total and subtotal hysterectomy, and be aware of which procedure your patient has had. It is important to know whether she needs to remain in the cervical screening programme or not.

Hysterectomy with bilateral salpingo-oophorectomy

Removal of the fallopian tubes and ovaries can be done at the same time as hysterectomy; this is known as hysterectomy with bilateral salpingo-oophorectomy. Benefits of this procedure are that the risk of ovarian cancer is removed, as is the risk of dyspareunia caused by ovaries adhering to the posterior fornix (although this should be avoided if the surgeon elevates the ovaries away from the pelvis). However, oophorectomy results in a sudden menopause if it had not already been reached, so hormone replacement therapy is often used to manage menopausal symptoms.

Surgical methods used to perform hysterectomy

There are a number of different ways in which the uterus can be accessed for removal.

- **Transvaginal hysterectomy** is preferred in most cases as it has a low morbidity, and quick postoperative recovery. This method is suitable for women with a mobile uterus that is no bigger than that equivalent to a 12-week pregnancy. Some surgeons see previous caesarean section as a contra-indication to vaginal hysterectomy, but certainly not all. Whether a vaginal hysterectomy can be tried after a caesarean section depends on how mobile the uterus feels and whether or not it is obviously stuck to the bladder.

- **Transabdominal hysterectomy** is reserved for those with a large bulky uterus (usually due to fibroids), and for cancer patients where pelvic node clearance is also required or direct visualisation of the pelvis recommended.

- **Laparoscopic hysterectomy** can be carried out using myolysis and embolisation techniques to break down uterine tissue, thus making pieces small enough to remove via a laparoscopic port.

Full recovery can take 1–2 weeks following laparoscopic or vaginal hysterectomy, and 6–8 weeks following abdominal hysterectomy. During this period, the woman should be advised to take plenty of rest and avoid heavy lifting. If it was an abdominal hysterectomy, she should see her practice nurse to check that the wound is healing adequately, and to have sutures removed if required. She should be advised not to drive a car until she is able to stamp her foot without feeling pain.

OOPHORECTOMY

Oophorectomy is the term used for removal of an ovary. Oophorectomy may be bilateral (removing both ovaries) or unilateral (removing just one ovary). Indications for oophorectomy include:

- Ovarian cancer.
- Prophylactic oophorectomy to prevent ovarian cancer in those of high risk, particularly for those women who carry BRCA1 or BRCA2 genes as oophorectomy results not only in removing the risk of ovarian cancer, but also significantly reduces the risk of developing a breast cancer.
- Large ovarian cysts.
- As an accompaniment to hysterectomy.

Hormone replacement following oophorectomy
The ovaries produce oestrogen, progesterone and testosterone, in various quantities, throughout a woman's life (not just in her fertile years). Oophorectomy results in a sudden withdrawal of this hormonal support, and a sudden menopause if the oophorectomy is performed before menopause was naturally reached. This sudden drop in hormone levels can be quite symptomatic and distressing. Hormone replacement therapy (HRT) is often prescribed to women who have not yet reached their natural menopause, to start straight after surgery, but it should be borne in mind that HRT does not fully compensate for the complete role of the ovaries, and symptoms can still occur.

Possible problems following oophorectomy
Following oophorectomy without subsequent HRT, there is an increased risk of cardiovascular disease (oestrogen is protective against ischaemic heart disease in women under 59 years old), osteopenia and fracture. Oophorectomy may also have an impact on sexuality, with possible reduction or elimination of libido and the inability to experience orgasm.

SALPINGECTOMY AND SALPINGOSTOMY

Salpingectomy is the term given to removal of a fallopian tube. As with oophorectomy, salpingectomy can be performed bilaterally with removal of both the tubes, or unilaterally with removal of just one tube. Indications for salpingectomy include ectopic pregnancy, hydrosalpinx and tubal cancer.

Salpingostomy is the term given to making an artificial opening in the fallopian tube; this procedure is carried out to remove an ectopic pregnancy, allowing preservation of the tube. This is important for future fertility, although it will increase the risk of a further ectopic pregnancy. Most procedures are performed laparoscopically, but some cases require open laparotomy.

LAPAROSCOPY

Laparoscopy involves the inspection and treatment of conditions in the abdominal cavity. It is done under anaesthetic; the abdominal cavity is insufflated with carbon dioxide to enable the organs to be seen, and a laparoscope is passed though a small incision in the abdominal wall.

Laparoscopy may be used for investigation (for example of suspected endometriosis) and for surgical procedures. Common examples of this are: tubal ligation, removal of endometriosis, management of ectopic pregnancy, myomectomy, removal of a perforated IUD, hysterectomy, and prolapse repair.

Contra-indications to laparoscopy include coagulation disorders and dense adhesions from previous abdominal surgery.

Women should be warned that they may have shoulder pain for a few days after their procedure; this is referred pain from the phrenic nerve. They should also be warned that complications such as injury to internal organs, or the inability to complete a process by laparoscopy, may mean that progression to open surgery may be required. Consent should be taken for this.

SURGICAL TREATMENTS FOR URINARY STRESS INCONTINENCE

TRANSVAGINAL TAPE

Insertion of a transvaginal tape is a urogynaecological treatment for urinary stress incontinence. The treatment involves the placement of a permanent synthetic mesh (known as the tension-free-tape) behind the urethra, which is then attached to the anterior abdominal wall. This tape then supports the urethra (Fig. 2.8).

Insertion of such tapes can be minimally invasive, requiring only very small incisions through the anterior vaginal wall to introduce the tape, and then small incisions in the anterior pelvis through which the trochars are removed. The operation may be performed under local or regional anaesthetic. If the patient is awake, it brings the advantage that the tension of the tape can be adjusted while the patient coughs. Insertion of a transvaginal tape has proved to be very successful in improving the symptoms of urinary stress incontinence.

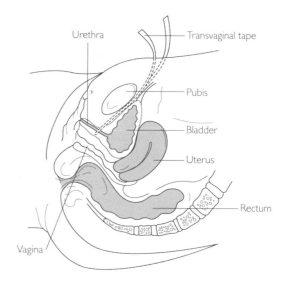

Figure 2.8 Diagram illustrating the use of the transvaginal tape procedure for treatment of urinary stress incontinence.

ANTERIOR COLPORRHAPHY

Anterior colporrhaphy is the term used for repair and refashioning of the anterior vaginal wall. It is the surgical treatment for prolapse of the bladder (cystocoele), urethra (urethrocoele) or both the bladder and urethra (cystourethrocoele). Anterior colporrhaphy involves incising the mucosa of the anterior wall of the vagina, fixing the bladder back into the correct position, and closing the trimmed mucosa to cover the repair.

POSTERIOR COLPORRHAPHY

Posterior colporrhaphy is the term used for repair and refashioning of the posterior vaginal wall. Posterior colporrhaphy is the surgical treatment for prolapse of the rectum (rectocoele). It involves incising the mucosa of the posterior wall of the vagina, fixing the rectum back into the correct position, and closing the trimmed mucosa to cover the repair.

COLPOSUSPENSION

Colposuspension literally means 'lifting of the vagina' and is another treatment for stress incontinence. It involves elevation of the paravesical tissue to the level of the ilio-inguinal ligament. It is less commonly performed now than the transvaginal tape procedure, as it requires a low transverse abdominal incision and a longer recovery, but is still seen as the gold standard for surgical stress incontinence management.

SACROCOLPOPEXY

Sacrocolpopexy is a surgical treatment for vault prolapse. It aims to lift the vagina back into its normal position. A synthetic mesh is used to support the vaginal vault by attachment to the sacral promontory. Sacrocolpopexy can be performed laparoscopically, or via a laparotomy abdominal incision (Fig. 2.9).

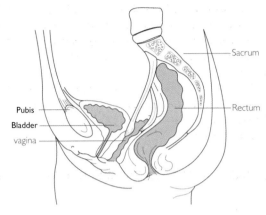

Figure 2.9 Sacrocolpopexy.

POSTOPERATIVE CARE

Following any vaginal wall repair procedure or insertion of a transvaginal tape, the woman should be advised to avoid sex for 6 weeks after the operation in order to allow adequate wound healing.

Module 3:
Antenatal care

You will be expected to understand and demonstrate appropriate knowledge and attitudes in relation to peri-conceptional care, antenatal care and maternal complications of pregnancy.

An awareness of substance misuse, psychiatric illness, problems of pregnancy at extremes of reproductive age and of domestic violence in relation to pregnancy is expected. An appreciation of emotional issues and cultural awareness is expected.

You will be expected to have a good understanding of common medical disorders and the effect that pregnancy may have on them, and also their effect, in turn, upon the pregnancy. A knowledge of therapeutics in antenatal care is expected. You will be expected to demonstrate your ability to assess and manage these conditions.

You will be expected to understand the principles of antenatal screening including screening for structural defects, chromosomal abnormalities and haemoglobinopathies and the effects upon fetus and neonate of relevant infections during pregnancy. You will need to show understanding of the roles of other professionals, the importance of liaison and empathic teamwork.

This is an important chapter. It explains thoroughly the care of pregnant women, from the time a couple presents for advice concerning conception, to confirming the pregnancy, routine scans and tests that are recommended, and how to manage pregnancies with complications. There is a lot of advice on the minor upsets that are common during pregnancy, and tips about simple ways to help. The interlinking roles of the midwives, GPs, obstetricians, the woman and her family are discussed.

USEFUL WEBSITE

- NICE Guidance: Antenatal care: routine care for the healthy pregnant woman
  <http://guidance.nice.org.uk/CG62>

THE ROLE OF THE MIDWIFE

The midwife provides continuity of care, looking after the woman throughout the pregnancy and often in subsequent pregnancies also. The midwife is generally the first port of call for women, offering an abundance of practical advice, support, and re-assurance.

ANTENATAL CHECK-UPS

The midwife will meet the woman and her partner (if involved) regularly throughout the pregnancy. A woman's schedule of antenatal appointments with her midwife will vary with the individual according to personal circumstance (*i.e.* more often if a teenager, socially isolated, learning disabled, or of clinically high risk) as well as local resources. The midwife is responsible for all the basic clinical tasks, such as monitoring the woman's blood pressure, checking her urine regularly for proteinuria and assessing the growth of the fetus by carrying out symphysis–fundal height measurements. As the pregnancy progresses, the midwife will discuss a birth plan, making suggestions on how best to prepare for labour. In addition, the midwife is a great source of helpful tips on managing the minor discomforts of pregnancy.

The midwife is responsible for performing 'booking bloods'. These are done early on in the pregnancy, and include a full blood count, rubella antibody titre, blood group and Rhesus status, hepatitis B, syphilis and HIV serology. It is recommended that 'at-risk groups' have a haemoglobinopathy screen.

The midwife will provide the pregnant woman with a pregnancy book, where all of her antenatal check-ups can be recorded. This book is kept by the woman herself. She is asked to bring it with her whenever she consults a healthcare professional, whether that is her midwife, GP, her obstetrician or an accident and emergency clinician. She should also be encouraged to take her pregnancy book with her whenever she travels, just in case she needs to use emergency services, or consult a GP out of her own area.

Assistance during labour

Every woman who delivers a baby in the UK has a right by law to be assisted throughout her labour by a qualified midwife. This is because it has been shown that one of the most important factors in determining a successful vaginal delivery is the presence of a midwife throughout the delivery process. This may or may not be the same midwife that looked after the woman during the pregnancy.

Care of the new mother and baby

The midwife is responsible for the mother and newborn baby for 10 days post-partum, extending to 28 days if necessary, at which point care is handed over to a health visitor. Midwives are responsible for teaching the pregnant woman how to breast-feed, and should encouraging this activity unless the mother is HIV positive, in which can breast-feeding is not recommended. Tuition in breast-feeding may be done on an individual basis, or more often as part of group antenatal classes.

The role of a midwife also includes provision of support for women following a late miscarriage or still-birth. Midwives can be a valuable source of support through what can be a very traumatic experience.

ROLE OF THE GENERAL PRACTITIONER

'BOOKING THE PREGNANCY'

The GP is often the first health professional to whom a woman presents once she suspects she may be pregnant. When this happens, the GP should confirm the pregnancy by performing a urinary pregnancy test if one has not already been done at home, enquire when the first day of the last menstrual period was, and estimate the gestation of the pregnancy. The role of the GP is then to assess whether this is a wanted or unwanted pregnancy and refer as appropriate. If the woman is pleased to be pregnant, the GP will refer her to the local antenatal provider. There is usually a degree of choice depending on the area; as such, some women may like to visit her local birthing units before making a choice on where they would prefer to deliver, and this idea can be offered.

MANAGING UNWANTED PREGNANCY

Should the pregnancy be unwanted, options available to the woman must be discussed:

- Continuing the pregnancy while working out ways to cope with a baby, for example, applying for child benefit, seeking help from local groups such as Sure Start, or seeking support from family members.

- Continuing pregnancy then after delivery giving the baby up for adoption.

- Terminating the pregnancy.

A rushed decision should never be made, and the patient should be encouraged to discuss her situation with a supportive friend, family member, or her partner. However, if there is any thought of a termination being wanted, an appointment should be booked (and cancelled if not wanted) as termination is far safer if carried out early.

CONTINUING CARE THROUGHOUT THE PREGNANCY

The GP also provides continuity of care; should any problems arise during pregnancy, the GP should be available to see the patient, either on a routine or urgent basis. There is usually close liaison between the midwife and the GP, so that medicines for simple ailments such as vaginal thrush can be easily accessed.

ROLE OF THE OBSTETRICIAN

Obstetrics (from the Latin word *obstare*, 'to stand by') is the surgical speciality that deals with the care of women and their babies during pregnancy, childbirth, and the puerperium. The obstetrician is based in secondary care and, as such, is less directly accessible to the patient. The obstetrician is generally only involved in antenatal care in complicated pregnancies where specialist input is required. Most pregnant women in the UK do not meet their obstetrician in the antenatal period, but may do so for the first time during labour, and certainly should they require a caesarean section. Many women, however, never meet their obstetrician as pregnancy, and delivery, takes place naturally without the need for any medical intervention. However, should there be any deviation from normal, or should problems develop during labour, the obstetrician is the source of expertise and, as such, will often play a large role in the care of the woman and her fetus.

It is the obstetrician who cares for women who develop complications during pregnancy and who, when indicated, performs assisted delivery of the fetus, whether that be vaginally or via caesarean section. The obstetrician is often involved in seeing women following miscarriage or still-birth, in addition to the GP who will continue to be the first port of call for the patient in the community once she has delivered.

LIFE-STYLE ADVICE

THE PLANNED PREGNANCY

It is a singular opportunity when a woman, or couple, visits the doctor or other healthcare professional for advice on pregnancy. It shows forethought and care by the future parents; planned pregnancies can help minimise complications developing. Preventative medicine is far more effective than reparative medicine. It is also a unique opportunity for a GP to build up a good relationship with the potential parents. For a couple, or single woman, to know that she has a healthcare professional, to whom she can come for advice, is of great value, particularly during this vulnerable time.

GOOD PRACTICE POINT 3.1

- When a woman comes to see you saying she would like to book in for pregnancy it is easy to give a lot of advice, take several measurements and fill-in an antenatal referral form. However, in your rush, do not forget to congratulate her on the good news, and establish rapport.

Preconception dietary advice

The woman can be advised to aim to achieve a body mass index (BMI) of 20–25 kg/m^2. To be of an ideal body weight not only optimises chances of conception, but also makes pregnancy more comfortable (there is more back pain, knee pain, and pelvic symphysis pain in overweight women). To be of ideal weight also decreases the likelihood of complications such as pre-eclampsia. A regular intake of fruit and vegetables is advised. Folic acid 400 mcg can be prescribed or bought over the counter, and ideally should be taken by the mother daily before starting to try for a baby and until 12 weeks' gestation, to help prevent neural tube defects (5 mg is needed where either partner has a family history of neural tube defects, if they have had a previous pregnancy affected by a neural tube defect, or if the woman has coeliac disease or other malabsorption state, diabetes mellitus, sickle-cell anaemia, or is taking antiepileptic medicines).

Preconception exercise

Exercise is encouraged for all women and their partners. A recommended schedule for this would be an aerobic exercise for approximately 20 minutes, three times weekly.

Smoking cessation pre-conception

If either partner smokes, then smoking cessation is encouraged. This can be achieved with the help of nicotine replacement products bought over the counter, or free from a primary care smoking cessation service. A new tablet, Varenicline (marketed as Champix), is also proving successful in supporting people trying to abandon their nicotine addiction. However, many smokers do break their habit simply by individual concentration and determination.

Cervical screening and sexual health pre-conception

Cervical screening is encouraged if such is due. Opportunistic testing for sexually transmitted infections is also encouraged.

Immune status pre-conception

Blood testing to discover the woman's immunity to rubella and varicella is recommended pre-conception. If tests show lack of immunity, vaccination should be offered. No other routine blood tests are required prior to conception.

Inherited disorders and genetic screening

One or both parents may have a family history of a genetic disorder. If this is the case, referral to a geneticist can help establish whether either parent does indeed carry a hereditary condition, and provide genetic counselling where necessary.

For common haemoglobinopathies, such as sickle cell anaemia and thalasaemia, diagnostic testing and advice can be provided in primary care. This is done by requesting a haemoglobinopathy screen.

General advice on how to conceive

Once a couple are ready to try for a baby, regular sexual intercourse (say three times a week) is the best way forward. The concentration of sexual activity to the ovulation period is practised successfully by some couples, although not generally advised due to the anxiety and stress it can cause. However, should couples meet only at infrequent intervals, then arranging sex to occur during the fertile time of the woman's menstrual cycle would be sensible.

ONCE PREGNANCY IS CONFIRMED

Once women miss a period and realise they are pregnant, they often visit their GP as a first port of call to ask for advice. This is particularly true for women experiencing their first pregnancy, or for those who have experienced problems in a previous pregnancy.

Suggested diet during pregnancy

What to eat is often a question pregnant women and their family ask their GP or family planning practitioner. Many women have cravings for particular foods during pregnancy, and these craving can be quite unusual, often being foods that the woman would not normally eat. As long as they do not contain anything harmful, the woman can be re-assured that this is nothing to worry about. All pregnant women should be advised to eat small meals often.

The diet of all pregnant women should contain a balance of carbohydrates, protein and roughage, and the UK Food Standards Agency recommends that pregnant women should all be encouraged to eat at least five portions of fruit or vegetables daily. Supplementation of the diet with 400 mcg of folic acid daily is recommended until the twelfth week of pregnancy. Current recommendations are complete cessation of alcohol, and to limit caffeine, and sugary foods.

Fermented cheeses such as camembert, stilton, and other live cheeses with rind should be avoided as they carry *Listeria* spp., as do all types of fresh paté. Meat should only be eaten if well cooked. Certain fish should be avoided altogether such as shark and swordfish (this is more important if you live in Iceland!), and tuna should be limited to two portions per week. This is because of the high levels of mercury in these fish which can compromise fetal neural development.

Sources of emotional support during pregnancy

It is important that pregnant women maintain good mental health through what can be an extremely tempestuous time. The most useful source of emotional support for many pregnant women is their partner, mother and friends. However, such support may be absent, or a source of stress and violence. In such situations, the GP and midwife are essential as a source of strength and encouragement. Support is often provided most effectively by a GP who is easily available for consultation, and who consistently provides a listening ear. Acknowledgement of her difficulties and alleviation of her concerns at each visit is important. Referral to local groups such as breast-feeding classes, antenatal groups, mother and baby meetings can also be of immense value.

With emotional issues, more than any other aspect of pregnancy care, treating the patient as an individual, with personal value systems and beliefs, is crucial. Although doctors are not expected to have much in-depth knowledge of the multitude of beliefs that exist, acknowledging that the patient holds such views can help establish rapport and trust between the doctor and patient. Many religious associations are able to provide support in their own cultural fashion, and knowledge of these groups by the GP, is often greatly appreciated.

THE BIRTH PLAN

Many antenatal clinics encourage a pregnant woman to consider the delivery of her baby, and how she would ideally like her labour to be managed. This can be written down, and is often referred to as 'the birth plan'. The formation of this plan is usually led by the midwife, who will discuss labour, current techniques and common practices. The midwife may also explore any fears or apprehensions the woman may have. It is important that birth plans are agreed to be an ideal, but it should be emphasized to the woman that a change of plan does not in any way indicate failure.

Place of delivery

Making a birth plan should include choosing a place for delivery. The choices are usually between delivery in an obstetric-led hospital labour ward, in a midwife-led birthing unit, or at home. The midwife would then go on to educate the woman on different positions of delivery, and the benefits of each. Birthing aids such as a birthing stool or birthing ball can be introduced, as can the idea of labouring and delivering in water. The midwife can take an opportunity, should one arise, to educate the woman regarding the benefits of moving around and changing positions frequently during labour to help descent of the baby through the birth canal. It is important to be aware of such factors when planning to deliver at home, for example, when re-arrangement of furniture, etc. may be beneficial.

Who will be present for the birth

The birth plan should also include who the woman would like to be present. Many labour wards only allow one birthing partner to be present, who in most cases will be the father or grandmother of the child, and this needs to be discussed prior to the event. If delivery is going to take place at home, as many friends and family members can be present as the woman would like.

Choice of analgesia

The birth plan should also give some thought as to what analgesia the woman would prefer; again, it is helpful if all the options are understood prior to the onset of labour. Written information can be supplied, and the woman may want to do her own research as there is a wealth of options available ranging from homeopathic drinks and aroma therapeutic candles, to Entonox, TENS machines, opioid injections and epidurals (see Module 4).

MINOR PREGNANCY COMPLICATIONS

There are a number of discomforts that a women may feel while pregnant. This section considers some of these common complaints, and suggests ways of dealing with them, so as to make pregnancy as enjoyable an experience for the mother as possible.

BACK PAIN

During pregnancy there are higher levels of circulating progesterone than usual. One of the actions of progesterone is to cause some joint laxity, important for allowing stretching of the pelvis during delivery. Joint laxity can, however, lead to back and hip pain during the pregnancy, and this is particularly apparent during the third trimester when the baby has become quite a heavy weight in the abdomen and pulls on the back. In some women, this is quite noticeable as an exaggerated lumbar spine lordosis. Sciatica may develop due to compression of the sciatic nerve; this can make it difficult for the pregnant woman to sit in any one position without experiencing pain.

Antenatal classes may provide advice on managing back pain, such as using appropriate back supports while sitting at work and while driving. Some women may find muscle rubs or hot baths helpful. Simple analgesia such as paracetamol can be taken regularly if required, and an opiate analgesic can be used if the pain is severe, such as co-dydramol or co-codamol, although these are likely to cause constipation. Physiotherapy is useful in the management of sciatica.

It is important that doctors take a careful history and examine women with back pain thoroughly, looking in particular for the development of any neurological symptoms or signs. Worrying signs would include new urinary or faecal incontinence, perineal numbness, gait disturbance, thoracic back pain, or focal bony tenderness. If any such signs are elicited, the woman should be referred to an accident and emergency department for further investigation, as it could be that nerve compression is developing which requires urgent surgical attention.

FATIGUE

Many women feel rather more tired than usual during pregnancy. This may be due to the higher metabolic rate, raised cardiac output, and generally rushed life of the pregnant woman. Women are often the main carers of a family unit, and the tiredness of a pregnant woman is easily exacerbated by any young children, elderly dependants or a spouse that she needs to look after, on top of the increased demands of caring for herself.

Iron-deficiency anaemia is common and, if present, will increase fatigue. It is recommended that if anaemia is present, ferrous sulphate dietary supplementation is taken, with advice to take measures to avoid constipation which may develop on such tablets.

VARICOSE VEINS

Due to increased pressure the fetus exerts in the pelvis, varicose veins can develop in the legs, vulva or vagina of pregnant women. These can be painful, especially if the complication of thrombophlebitis or vascular thrombosis develops. Elasticated stockings, rest, and raising legs on a stool are all suggested treatments. Some women find topical Heparinoid cream 0.3% soothing.

If varicose veins persist longer than 3 months' post-partum, consultation with a vascular surgeon is recommended for venous stripping or sclerosal venous injection.

CONSTIPATION

Straining at stool is discouraged during pregnancy, especially in the third trimester, as straining predisposes to the development of haemorrhoids (see below). Pregnant women are, therefore, encouraged to eat a diet high in fibre.

If dietary and life-style changes fail to control constipation in pregnancy, a bulk-forming laxative such as Ispaghula husk is recommended as a first-line treatment. Lactulose is safe in pregnancy, but must be used with caution in the diabetic woman. Senna is also safe during pregnancy, but it is a stimulant laxative and so may result in abdominal cramps, causing concern to a pregnant woman.

HAEMORRHOIDS

Haemorrhoids (also known as piles) are a common ailment of pregnant women. Haemorrhoids are dilated vascular cushions that can protrude from the anus, bleed and cause pain when straining at stool. Haemorrhoids are worsened by constipation, and compounded by the pressure of the fetus in the pelvis during pregnancy. Haemorrhoids may also be exacerbated by the pressure of the fetus moving through the birth canal during vaginal delivery.

The symptoms of haemorrhoids can be minimised by avoiding constipation. Topical ointments such as Anusol and rectal suppositories such as Proctosedyl are available to purchase over the counter, or can be prescribed. These contain a mild steroid with a topical anaesthetic and antiseptic, and provide good relief. In many cases, haemorrhoids improve considerably in the 3 months following delivery, and referral to a surgeon for consideration of banding or haemorrhoidectomy should be delayed until then if symptoms persist.

INSOMNIA

Insomnia is commonly experienced by expectant mothers due to fetal movement, and a general difficulty finding a comfortable sleeping position due to the weight of the fetus in the abdomen.

Sedating drugs are not recommended, and management is based on re-assurance and relaxing techniques. Women should be advised not to lie on their backs during the third trimester as this compresses the inferior vena cava, thus compromising venous return to the heart.

BLOATING AND ACID REFLUX

Bloating is a common symptom of early pregnancy. Re-assurance is usually all that is required. Acid reflux is a common symptom of late pregnancy. It is caused by laxity of the lower oesophageal sphincter, as well as the physical presence of the fetus pressing on and kicking the stomach. The condition is more troublesome in smokers, women with high alcohol consumption, those with known peptic ulcer disease, or *Helicobacter pylori* infection.

Advice to pregnant women experiencing bloating and/or reflux is to eat small amounts often, and to avoid spicy and other irritant foods, large heavy meals, and alcohol. Sleeping propped up on pillows, and taking Gaviscon as and when required is often helpful.

HYPEREMESIS GRAVIDARUM

Nausea is common throughout pregnancy, but particularly in the first trimester, peaking in severity at approximately 10 weeks' gestation. Hyperemesis gravidarum is the Latin term given to describe the excessive vomiting that can occur during pregnancy. Hyperemesis gravidarum can be more severe in pregnancies of multiple gestation or a hydatidiform mole. As such, patients with hyperemesis should have a scan to exclude twins or a molar pregnancy.

Advice is to eat small amounts often, and a tip from the midwives is to nibble on ginger biscuits. Prochlorperazine can be administered orally, rectally or as buccal tablets. If prochlorperizine is ineffective, an oral preparation of metoclopramide and/or cyclizine can be added. Patients who are unable to keep anything down by mouth may require admission to hospital for intravenous fluid rehydration and intravenous anti-emetics. Signs of severe hyperemesis, which requires hospital admission, are the presence of ketones in the urine, and a raised serum urea.

PRURITIS GRAVIDARUM

Generalised pruritis is a common phenomenon of late pregnancy. Liver function tests can be checked to exclude obstetric cholestasis; more often than not, no cause is found. Recommended treatment is the application of topical aqueous cream with 2% menthol, ideally kept in the fridge. Antihistamines will lessen the itch but will make both mother and baby drowsy, and so are usually avoided. The condition resolves following delivery, but recurs in up to half of subsequent pregnancies.

OBSTETRIC CHOLESTASIS

Obstetric cholestasis is also known as intrahepatic cholestasis of pregnancy, and occurs in about 1% of pregnancies, being more common in multiple pregnancy. Obstetric cholestasis is due to stasis and build up of bile within the hepatic biliary ducts, and is multifactorial. The condition usually occurs in the third trimester of pregnancy, and resolves after delivery, but can be a cause of premature labour and intra-uterine death.

Obstetric cholestasis can cause generalised pruritis without any rash (pruritis gravidarium), mild jaundice, nausea and fatigue. Itching is most severe on the palms of the hands and the soles of the feet. The intense itch can be very uncomfortable, and is particularly bad at night, which prevents sleep. Liver function tests are abnormal with raised aspartate transaminase (AST), alanine transaminase (ALT) and gamma-glutamyl transpeptidase (γ-GT). The chief diagnostic test is a rise in bile acid levels, though not all units offer this test. Bilirubin is often within the normal range, but may be raised. If bilirubin is raised, and there are light stools and dark urine, gallstones need to be excluded as a cause. All women should undergo testing for viral hepatitis and receive an ultrasound scan of the liver to exclude other causes of abnormal liver function tests before accepting the diagnosis of obstetric cholestasis.

Treatment of obstetric cholestasis involves topical emollients and oral antihistamines for symptomatic relief. Ursodeoxycholic acid is helpful in reducing itch, but does not reduce the fetal complication risk. Many obstetricians recommend induction of labour for women affected by obstetric cholestasis at 37–38 weeks' gestation. Women are offered oral vitamin K at a dose of 10 mg daily to minimise the chance of post-partum and neonatal bleeding.

RED DEGENERATION OF FIBROIDS

Uterine fibroids are common, particularly among older women of African or Caribbean origin; during pregnancy, fibroids can be the cause of considerable pain. Fibroids are made of smooth muscle, and demand a large blood supply, which becomes a problem during pregnancy as blood supply to a growing fibroid may be unable to keep pace with the more pressing demand for blood and oxygen from the growing fetus. This causes degeneration of the fibroid, which turns red as it becomes ischaemic. The resulting fibroid mass becomes a source of severe pain.

Pain from red degeneration of fibroids can be managed with paracetamol or a mild opiate as necessary. Non-steroidal anti-inflammatory drugs (NSAIDs), such as ibuprofen and diclofenac, should be avoided in pregnancy as they can cause closure of the fetal ductus arteriosus, and possibly persistent pulmonary hypertension of the newborn. NSAIDs are also associated with delayed onset and increased duration of labour. If the pain from red degeneration is extreme, hospital admission may be required for intravenous opiate analgesia and fluids. Extreme pain can precipitate uterine contractions, but this is rare.

URINARY FREQUENCY

Sometimes, the first symptom of pregnancy that a woman notices is urinary frequency. This is a direct consequence of the pregnant uterus lying on the bladder. By late pregnancy, most women are woken at least once each night to urinate, and many women may wake even more frequently. This is normal, and re-assurance can be given.

Urinary tract infection is another cause of urinary frequency but although common, is not normal, and requires treatment (see below).

SERIOUS PREGNANCY COMPLICATIONS

INTRA-UTERINE GROWTH RESTRICTION

Intra-uterine growth restriction (IUGR) is the term given to the condition when the fetus is not reaching its full growth potential, and becomes small for its gestational age. This is generally taken to be when the abdominal circumference is smaller than the fifth centile. However, it should be remembered that a fetus can be growth restricted and still have an abdominal circumference greater than the fifth centile. The important point is to see the centile of the head circumference in relation to the abdominal circumference; a growth-restricted fetus will exhibit head-sparing until the situation is extremely severe. Some fetuses are, however, small for their gestational age due to constitutionally small parents. This is a normal variant, and separate to IUGR; IUGR is always pathological.

Symmetrically growth-restricted fetuses (those with a small body and small sized head to match) are usually a result of intrinsic problem with the fetus or a maternal condition. Asymmetrically growth-restricted fetuses (those with a small body but normal-sized head) are usually a result of placental insufficiency.

Maternal causes of IUGR

Common maternal causes of intra-uterine growth restriction include:

- Malnutrition (the most common cause of IUGR world-wide).
- Smoking or illicit drug abuse.
- Viral infection, such as cytomegalovirus, rubella, or toxoplasmosis infection.
- Chronic maternal disease such as hypertension, cyanotic heart disease, respiratory disease, sickle cell anaemia, anti-phospholipid syndrome.

Fetal causes of IUGR

Common fetal causes of intra-uterine growth restriction include: chromosomal abnormality and multiple gestation. It is important that the midwife and GP are able to detect IUGR, as early referral to an obstetrician can make a vast difference to the prognosis. In general, if, on examining the pregnant woman, the distance between the symphysis pubis and the uterine fundus is found to be 3 cm less than expected according to dates, referral should be made.

GOOD PRACTICE POINT 3.2

- If the symphysis-fundal height is > 3 cm less than expected according to dates, this may indicate intra-uterine growth restriction which needs urgent referral to the obstetrician for ultrasound scanning.

Treatment of IUGR

Once IUGR has been recognised, weekly Doppler ultrasound scans are carried out to monitor fetal growth, and assess flow of blood through the umbilical artery. If the growth restriction becomes critical and umbilical blood flow poor, pre-term delivery by elective caesarean section may be offered. IUGR can result in intra-uterine death if the condition continues without intervention.

PLACENTA PRAEVIA

Placenta praevia is the term given to the situation when the placenta is sited in the lower uterine segment. It is diagnosed on ultrasound scan.

In partial placenta praevia, the placenta partially covers the cervical os, but the fetus should be able to pass the placenta to enter the birth canal once the cervix has dilated. In complete placenta praevia, the placenta completely

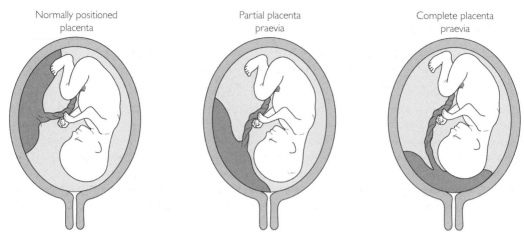

Normally positioned placenta | Partial placenta praevia | Complete placenta praevia

Figure 3.1 Placenta praevia.

obstructs the cervical os, even when the cervix is dilated, and the fetus is unable to navigate past it (Fig. 3.1).

Placenta praevia is more common in women carrying multiple gestation pregnancies, women who have undergone a previous caesarean section, or who have uterine cavity distortion for any reason.

Symptoms and signs of placenta praevia

Placenta praevia typically presents as painless vaginal bleeding during the second or third trimester. The bleeding is from the maternal circulation, not from the fetus and, as such, results in maternal compromise. If bleeding is mild to moderate, the management is conservative. If bleeding is severe, and especially if the mother is showing signs of shock, emergency referral to labour ward is necessary, for maternal resuscitation and consideration of emergency delivery.

Placenta accreta

Placenta accreta is a rare condition where the placenta erodes through the uterine wall, and usually occurs when the placenta implants over a previous caesarean section scar. It is different from placenta praevia.

GOOD PRACTICE POINT 3.3

- It is dangerous to perform a vaginal examination if there is placenta praevia.
  Examination can cause a torrential, and fatal, haemorrhage and so should never be done.

PRE-ECLAMPSIA

Pre-eclampsia is a multisystem disorder specific to pregnancy. It is a result of maternal vascular endothelial activation (the cause of which still remains unknown), which leads to generalised vasospasm, increased systemic vascular resistance, platelet activation and the development of a highly coagulable state. There is usually hypertension, proteinuria, peripheral and pulmonary oedema. The mother may suffer a deep vein thrombosis, pulmonary embolism, renal artery thrombosis or stroke.

Risk factors for development of pre-eclampsia

Risk factors for the development of pre-eclampsia include first pregnancy, pre-existing hypertension, renal disease, diabetes, multiple pregnancy, and anti-phospholipid syndrome. A new partner confers a risk similar to that of a primipara.

> **GOOD PRACTICE POINT 3.4**
>
> - Blood pressure should be checked regularly in all pregnant woman. If it is found to be high, the urine should be checked for protein. If proteinuria is found, the woman should be referred immediately to the labour ward or antenatal clinic for observation and 24-hour urine collection.

Symptoms and signs of pre-eclampsia

Symptoms of pre-eclampsia include: (i) headache and blurred vision; (ii) epigastric/upper abdominal pain; and (iii) nausea and vomiting.

Signs of pre-eclampsia include: (i) hypertension (blood pressure is over 140/90); (ii) proteinuria (24-hour urine collection protein > 3 g); (iii) brisk reflexes; (iv) ankle clonus; (v) wide-spread oedema; and (vi) intra-uterine growth retardation.

Treatment of pre-eclampsia

Any pregnant woman with pre-eclampsia must be monitored extremely closely. This may require daily visits to the day-pregnancy unit, or even admission to labour ward, particularly if neurological signs are developing. The blood pressure is controlled by the administration of antihypertensives such as methyl-dopa and/or labetalol. Most clinicians will treat blood pressure levels greater than 140/90. If pre-eclampsia presents during labour, the blood pressure can be lowered by the use of intravenous hydralazine and/or epidural anaesthesia. Strict fluid balance and monitoring of renal function is vitally important. Magnesium sulphate is given if there is hyper-reflexia associated with hypertension, and is used to treat eclampsia as well as to prevent further convulsions.

Delivery of the fetus is the only curative treatment for pre-eclampsia, and the decision as to when to deliver needs to be made by the patient under the advice of an obstetrician as well as a neonatologist. The baby will be compromised if delivered pre-term, but early delivery may be the only way to preserve the life of the mother.

After delivery, the blood pressure usually returns to normal within a couple of weeks. The new mother is usually discharged from the maternity ward on labetalol and/or methyldopa. The GP would be expected to monitor the use of this, and slowly stop the anti-hypertensive agent when appropriate, which is usually within a couple of weeks of the delivery. Occasionally long-term blood pressure control will be required, and the GP should manage that in the usual way.

> **USEFUL WEBSITE**
>
> - Action on pre-eclampsia <http://www.apec.org.uk/>

ECLAMPSIA

Eclampsia is a grand mal convulsion occurring in association with pre-eclampsia, but may arise before the development of hypertension and proteinuria. Eclamptic fits can occur before, during or after delivery. Eclampsia can be fatal.

HELLP

Haemolysis, elevated liver enzymes, low platelets (HELLP) is a particularly severe form of pre-eclampsia, affecting 5% of pre-eclampsia sufferers, and is an obstetric emergency. There is high risk of fetal loss due to placental abruption, and a high risk of maternal death due to disseminated intravascular coagulation and acute renal failure.

PREMATURE RUPTURE OF MEMBRANES

Premature rupture of membranes (PROM) refers to the rupture of the amniotic membrane between 24–37 weeks' gestation. PROM may be precipitated by vaginal infection such as bacterial vaginosis.

Symptoms of premature rupture of membranes

Some women experiencing PROM describe a gush of water from the vagina, others describe slow leakage of clear fluid noticed only due to the discovery of damp underwear. The woman may or may not notice decreased fetal movements. An ultrasound scan usually shows oligohydramnios due to loss of amniotic fluid, but this is not diagnostic of PROM in itself. Diagnosis of PROM must be confirmed by sterile speculum examination that demonstrates amniotic fluid pooling in the posterior vagina. The cervix should also be visualised, in order to assess whether dilatation has begun.

Management of premature rupture of membranes

Any woman with confirmed PROM should have some blood tests taken, including a full blood count, C-reactive protein and a sample taken for 'group and save' in case blood transfusion becomes necessary. Fetal cardiotocography (CTG) monitoring is often used, but an ultrasound scan is only performed if justified for other reasons. Vaginal swabs should be taken for microscopy, culture and sensitivity. Prophylactic penicillin or erythromycin is usually administered.

GOOD PRACTICE POINT 3.5

- Of all PROM cases, 50% lead to premature onset of labour. As a result, it is considered good practice to offer betamethasone to promote fetal lung production of surfactant.

- Tocolytics are contra-indicated; if infection is developing and labour is prevented, both the mother and fetus may become septic.

When a woman gives a history suggestive of premature rupture of membranes, do not examine the woman in your GP surgery; the fewer speculum examinations she has the better, so as to minimise risk of infection. Referral should be made directly to the labour ward, and she can be examined there. Remember a premature delivery may be imminent.

MATERNAL INFECTION DURING PREGNANCY

All living things are susceptible to infections of one sort or another and pregnant women are no exception. There are a number of infections that cause particular concern during pregnancy, and this section will address these. Sexually transmitted infections are discussed in detail in Module 6, but are mentioned here in the context of pregnancy.

HIV INFECTION IN PREGNANCY

HIV has three main mechanisms of transmission:

- Sexual transmission during unprotected penetrative anal, vaginal, or rarely oral intercourse.
- Vertical transmission between mother and child.
- Blood-borne transmission via transfusion of infected blood products, either medically from a contaminated a blood transfusion, accidentally such as by needle stick injury, or carelessly from the use of shared needles in recreational drug abuse.

Women with HIV are at a small increased risk of adverse pregnancy outcomes such as spontaneous abortion, still-birth and intra-uterine growth retardation. If the baby is born with HIV, it will be at risk of developing AIDS and dying in childhood unless antiretroviral medication is taken throughout life.

HIV testing

As HIV can be carried asymptomatically for a number of years, all women in the UK are routinely offered HIV testing during the first trimester of pregnancy, using an 'opt-out' rather than 'opt-in' system, so that HIV-positive women can be identified and action can be taken to prevent the mother transmitting the virus to her unborn child.

GOOD PRACTICE POINTS 3.6

- All GPs are likely at some point in their career to have to tell someone the news that they are HIV positive. Be prepared for this. Know where your local HIV services are. Ensure the patient is safe, and has somewhere to go when they leave your consultation room. Ensure they understand the importance of informing their sexual partner. Repeat the HIV test to confirm the result. Arrange to see them again soon.

HIV treatment to the mother and newborn

If maternal HIV infection is detected, modern antiretroviral agents (usually zidovudine or AZT) are offered to the mother from 24 weeks' gestation, and given to the neonate during the first 6 weeks of life. With this regimen, combined with an elective caesarean section and avoidance of breast feeding, HIV transmission from mother to baby is successfully prevented in over 98% of cases. If no preventative measures are taken, transmission of HIV infection from the mother to the neonate is approximately 40%.

CHLAMYDIAL INFECTION IN PREGNANCY

If a mother is infected with chlamydia at the time of delivery, transmission to the fetus can occur as it passes through the birth canal. This may cause neonatal eye infection (ophthalmia neonatorum) and neonatal pneumonitis.

As chlamydial infection is often asymptomatic, pregnant women carrying *Chlamydia trachomatis* may only discover they are infected when their neonate develops clinical disease. In areas of the UK with very high prevalence, screening for vaginal chlamydial infection may be routinely offered to pregnant women. Opportunistic screening is also encouraged by all GP surgeries and sexual health clinics.

Treatment of chlamydia in pregnancy

Treatment of chlamydia in pregnancy currently consists of Azithromycin 1 g stat (with partner notification and abstinence until a week after all concerned are treated). Azithromycin is not actually licenced for use in pregnancy, but is used successfully in many gastro-urinary clinics where it has been found to be more effective than the alternative regimen of 2 weeks of erythromycin 500 mg bd.

Doxycycline should be avoided in pregnancy and breast feeding.

GONORRHOEAL INFECTION IN PREGNANCY

As with chlamydia, maternal vaginal infection with gonorrhoea can be passed to the fetus as it passes through the birth canal. This may result in ophthalmia neonatorum, and will present with a red eye a few days after birth, which can develop into a pan-ophthalmitis that results in blindness within 24 hours.

Both chlamydia and gonorrhoea infection can precipitate pre-term delivery.

Treatment of gonorrhoea in pregnancy

Treatment of gonorrhoea in pregnancy is currently with cefixime 400 mg stat. If the diagnosis is made on a NAATs test, it is essential that a charcoal swab is taken at the time of treatment to check antibiotic sensitivities. The woman will then need to be recalled for an alternative antibiotic if she is found to carry a resistant strain.

GENITAL HERPES IN PREGNANCY

Genital herpes is a sexually transmitted infection caused by the herpes simplex virus. It presents with recurrent outbreaks of painful genital ulcers in the mother. Very rarely, the fetus can be systemically infected; this causes low birth weight, and premature delivery. The baby will then suffer from neonatal herpes.

Neonatal herpes

Neonatal herpes infection is a rare, but serious, condition caused by vertical transmission from an infected mother to the fetus during child-birth. It is most likely to occur when the mother acquired a primary herpes infection during the third trimester of pregnancy.

Neonatal herpes can affect the skin of the baby, causing ulceration. Lesions typically appear on sites of trauma such as the attachment sites of fetal scalp electrodes, forceps or vacuum extractors, or at the base of the glans penis following circumcision. The orbits or nasopharynx of the neonate may also be involved.

It is rare, but a neonate can develop disseminated herpes, with viral septicaemia, encephalitis and hepatic failure. Such a baby will present with seizures, tremor, irritability, and a bulging fontanelle. There is a high morbidity and mortality in such cases.

Treatment of genital herpes in pregnancy

To prevent neonatal herpes infection, women with their first attack of genital herpes ulceration at the time of delivery should have an elective caesarean section. Women with known herpes, but without genital ulceration, can deliver vaginally and may be offered prophylactic acyclovir, which is safe during pregnancy.

GENITAL WARTS IN PREGNANCY

Genital warts may appear for the first time in pregnancy due to the changes in the woman's immune system rather than recent exposure to the virus, and the GP should explain this. Genital warts that were previously present, may enlarge during the pregnancy, but the lady can be re-assured that they generally vanish shortly after delivery.

Treatment of genital warts in pregnancy

Treatment aims to reduce the exposure of the baby to the human papilloma virus, but podophyllin, podophyllotxin and 5-fluorouracil are teratogenic and must not be used. Imiqimod is not licenced for use in pregnancy and should also be avoided.

The fetus may pick up the virus during its navigation through the birth canal; very occasionally, development of laryngeal papillomatosis or anogenital warts are seen in the neonate as a result of this. Because of the rarity of this event, caesarean section is not indicated.

SYPHILIS IN PREGNANCY

All pregnant women are screened for syphilis as congenital syphilis is a serious condition which needs to be diagnosed if present. Congenital syphilis can result in permanent and severe skeletal and neurological abnormalities in the neonate, as well as congenital deafness. Still-birth and perinatal death can also occur.

It is essential that any blood tests positive for syphilis are interpreted by an expert (see Module 6 for the blood tests used in diagnosis). Non-specific tests may give a false-positive result for a number of reasons, including pregnancy itself and, rarely, a different, non-sexually transmitted, treponemal infection (such as Yaws, Pinta or Bejel) which also occur in the UK . Great distress and damage to the woman's relationship may be caused if a wrong diagnosis is given.

HEPATITIS B IN PREGNANCY

If the mother is a carrier of hepatitis B, and especially should she be HepB e-antigen positive (which indicates high infectivity), consent for immunisation of the neonate should be obtained during pregnancy so that active and passive immunisation can be given to the neonate immediately after birth. Breast feeding is not contra-indicated.

BACTERIAL VAGINOSIS IN PREGNANCY

Bacterial vaginosis, as described in Module 1, is associated with overgrowth of anaerobic vaginal flora, causing an offensive vaginal discharge with a characteristic smell. When present during the third trimester of pregnancy, bacterial vaginosis can precipitate pre-term delivery of the fetus.

Treatment is with metronidazole 400 mg bd for 5 days. It is recommended that high-dose regimens of metronidazole such as 2 g stat should be avoided in pregnancy.

GROUP B STREPTOCOCCUS INFECTION IN PREGNANCY

Group B streptococcus (GBS) is a Gram-positive coccus characterised by the presence of Group B Lancefield antigen. It is also known as *Streptococcus agalactiae*. GBS is a member of the normal flora of the gut and female urogenital tract, and does no harm. It is carried by at least a quarter of all women, and infection with GBS can come and go.

As the fetus passes through the birth canal of an infected mother, it is quite likely to come into contact with GBS, and become colonised with it. The vast majority of babies are unaffected by this, but a small number can become seriously ill.

Testing for group B streptococcus

In many countries, including the USA, Canada and Australia, all women are routinely tested for group B streptococcus by swabbing the vagina and rectum during the 36th week of pregnancy, and the mother is treated with penicillin (or clindamycin if penicillin-allergic) if she is found to be a carrier.

In the UK, routine testing in this way is thought to be neither good practice nor cost effective, as there is a very low risk associated with most cases of GBS carriage. A positive result in most cases would only result in unnecessary and potentially harmful treatment; only 1 in 500 babies born to mothers with a positive test are likely to develop a GBS infection. In addition, a negative swab result taken from the mother 2 weeks prior to delivery, does not guarantee that she will not be a GBS carrier at the time of delivery.

Treatment of group B streptococcus

The Royal College of Obstetricians and Gynaecologists advises giving antibiotics to: (i) all women with prolonged rupture of membranes; (ii) all women with a temperature of 38°C or more; and (iii) all women in preterm labour.

Neonatal GBS infection

A baby infected with group B streptococcus can develop pneumonia, meningitis and septicaemia, all of which carry high morbidity and mortality. All neonates at risk are, therefore, carefully observed for the first 24–48 hours, and treated with antibiotics if any sign of infection develops.

LISTERIA INFECTION IN PREGNANCY

Listeria monocytogenes is an aerobic and facultative anaerobic, Gram-positive rod found in soil and water. Many animals carry the bacterium asymptomatically, and many vegetables are colonised from the soil or from manure used as fertilizer. Because of this, *Listeria* is found in a variety of raw foods, such as uncooked meats and vegetables, as well as in processed foods that become contaminated after processing such as cold cuts and fresh cheeses. Unpasteurised milk may also contain the bacterium.

Listeriosis

Listeriosis is an infection developed following eating food containing *L monocytogenes* in susceptible individuals. The disease primarily affects pregnant women, newborns, and immunosuppressed adults. Infected pregnant women may experience only a mild, flu-like illness, but the infection can lead to miscarriage, premature delivery, or still-birth. In the neonate, infection may result in septicaemia.

Pregnant women are advised to drink only pasteurised milk and cheeses, to cook meat well, and to wash vegetables thoroughly before consuming.

Treatment of listeriosis

Treatment of listeriosis is with intravenous ampicillin and gentamicin.

MALARIAL INFECTION DURING PREGNANCY

Malaria is caused by a protozoan parasite *Plasmodium*, which is transmitted by the bite of the female anopheline mosquito. Malaria can only, therefore, be caught where the anopheline mosquito lives; this is most of sub-Saharan Africa, South America, and South-East Asia. Malaria cannot be contracted in the UK, but malaria does affect the UK population as they are exposed to the disease when they travel abroad.

Pregnant women are more vulnerable to malaria than other adults, particularly during the first trimester of pregnancy when they are four times more likely to get malaria than other adults, and twice as likely to die of it. Malaria can be quite deceptive; when only a few parasites can be detected in blood, the placenta may be heavily infected. The effects are worse if it is the woman's first pregnancy, and if she has no prior malaria immunity (typically the Western tourist on holiday, or an African native returning home after being in the West for a number of years).

Symptoms of malaria

Malaria is characterised by intermittent high fever, severe headache, and profound malaise causing prostration. *Falciparum* malaria causes red cell destruction, which can lead on to a severe anaemia, splenomegaly, renal failure, convulsions, sepsis, coma and even death of both mother and child.

Diagnosing malaria

Malaria is tested for by visualising the parasite on thick and thin blood films.

Malaria prevention

Prophylaxis is recommended to any individual travelling to a country where malaria is endemic. There are a number of drugs available for this; however, due to increasing drug resistance, prophylaxis is not fully effective and infection can still occur.

A number of malaria prophylactic agents are contra-indicated during pregnancy, such as malarone and doxycycline. Chloroquine and proguanil are safe in pregnancy, but are not so effective in preventing malaria. For this reason, advice is that travel to endemic malarial areas should be avoided during pregnancy if at all possible. If travel is essential, emphasis is made to avoid mosquito bites. The suggested way of doing this is by the use of insect repellents containing diethyltoluamide (DEET), bed-nets soaked in permethrin, the wearing long clothes, and staying indoors at dusk. These methods are all safe during pregnancy and breast-feeding.

RUBELLA DURING PREGNANCY

Rubella is caused by an RNA virus, which causes a mild, self-limiting, febrile illness associated with development of a macular rash and lymphadenopathy.

Congenital rubella syndrome

If primary maternal infection occurs during pregnancy, it can result in miscarriage, particularly if infection is in the first trimester. If the fetus survives, it is likely to suffer from congenital rubella syndrome. This entails:

- Sensorineural deafness in 80%. Rubella is the most common cause of congenital deafness in the developed world.
- Severe learning difficulty in 55%.
- Insulin-dependent diabetes in 20%.
- Congenital heart defects.
- A range of eye defects, including cataract and congenital glaucoma.

Prevention of rubella

Rubella is now a rare illness due to the introduction of the measles, mumps, rubella (MMR) vaccine into the immunisation schedule of all children in the UK. However, occasional cases of rubella do sometimes occur, usually in unvaccinated children.

All pregnant women should be tested to see whether they have immunity to rubella. If they are found to lack immunity, it is important that they avoid any children (or indeed adults) with febrile illnesses and rash during their pregnancy. Such women will be offered rubella vaccination soon after delivery.

Treatment of rubella

There is no treatment for rubella infection, or congenital rubella syndrome, so the aim is to prevent infection.

TOXOPLASMOSIS DURING PREGNANCY

Toxoplasmosis is caused by the intracellular parasite *Toxoplasma gondii*. Cats are the main source of infection. Infectious cysts are excreted by cats for up to 2 weeks after their initial infection, and these cysts can survive in warm, moist soil for more than a year. Humans can acquire the infection from dealing with cat litter, or from eating raw or undercooked meat of an intermediate host. For these reasons, it is recommended that pregnant women avoid contact with cat litter, wear gloves when gardening and during any contact with soil or sand, and only eat well-cooked meat.

Pregnant women with toxoplasmosis may be asymptomatic, or suffer a mild flu-like illness which is rarely severe. However, toxoplasmosis is an important illness as it can cause miscarriage if infection takes place close to conception. The chance of infection increases as the pregnancy proceeds, but the consequences become less severe.

Complications of toxoplasmosis

If the fetus becomes infected with toxoplasmosis, a classic triad of chorioretinitis, intracranial calcification, and hydrocephalus is seen. Congenital toxoplasmosis is very rare.

URINARY TRACT INFECTION IN PREGNANCY

Urinary tract infection is very common among sexually active women, and becomes even more common in pregnancy due to the slightly immunocompromised state of the pregnant woman, and the distortion of her urinary bladder. Urinary tract infection usually presents with dysuria, urinary frequency and urgency, and sometimes pelvic pain and fever. A mid-stream urine sample should be taken, tested with a urine dipstick, and if positive for leukocytes, nitrite or protein sent to the laboratory for microscopy, culture and sensitivity.

Antibiotic treatment of urinary tract infection in pregnancy

Until the laboratory results are back, first-line antibiotics recommended for the treatment of urinary tract infection in pregnancy are: cephalexin 500 mg bd for 3 days, amoxicillin 250 mg tds for 5 days, or erythromycin 500 mg bd for 5 days. Once bacterial culture and antibiotic sensitivities are available (it usually takes at least 48 hours for the laboratory to grow the bacteria sufficiently enough to produce a report), the antibiotic treatment can be changed as appropriate.

General advice is that, in addition to the antibiotics, the woman should drink plenty of clear fluids and rest until symptoms improve. Simple analgesia such as paracetamol can be taken.

Antibiotics contra-indicated during pregnancy

Trimethoprim is contra-indicated as it is a folate antagonist that will compromise fetal neural development. Nitrofurantoin is contra-indicated during the third trimester of pregnancy as it is associated with neonatal haemolysis if used close to delivery time. Also contra-indicated in pregnancy are ciprofloxacin, norfloxacin, tetracycline, chloramphenicol and aminoglycosides.

GOOD PRACTICE POINTS 3.7

- There is an excellent section in the back of the *BNF*, Appendix 4, which lists drugs and their safety profile in pregnancy. Always consult this before prescribing to a pregnant woman.

VARICELLA ZOSTER INFECTION DURING PREGNANCY

The varicella zoster virus causes chickenpox on primary infection, and shingles on re-activation. The varicella zoster virus is very highly contagious; it is airborne, and can be caught by simply being in the same room as an infected individual.

Chickenpox is usually a mild, self-limiting, febrile illness of childhood characterised by a wide-spread vesicular rash. However, if a woman catches chickenpox for the first time during her pregnancy, she can become very unwell indeed, developing pneumonitis and/or encephalitis.

Congenital varicella syndrome

If chickenpox is caught by the pregnant woman in the first or second trimester of pregnancy, 2% of fetuses will develop congenital varicella syndrome. The extent to which the fetus is affected is not related to the severity of disease in the mother.

Signs of congenital varicella syndrome include: (i) intra-uterine growth retardation; (ii) microcephaly with cortical atrophy; (iii) limb hypoplasia; (iv) microphthalmia, cataracts and chorioretinitis; and (v) deafness.

Varicella infection during the third trimester

If maternal varicella infection occurs in the third trimester, there is no adverse effect on the fetus. However, if the mother is infected by varicella at the time of delivery, both mother and baby may be affected by a severe and life-threatening chickenpox infection with long-lasting effects.

SCREENING

ANTENATAL SCREENING

Antenatal screening is a way of assessing whether a fetus has an abnormality or medical condition. Antenatal screening has three main aims:

- To give the parents the chance to abort a fetus with a diagnosed abnormal condition, such as Down's syndrome.
- To enable timely medical or surgical treatment of a condition before and after birth, such as fetal cardiac surgery.
- To give parents and the healthcare team the chance to prepare to deliver a baby with a health problem or disability, and to prepare for the possibility of a still-birth.

Initial screening tests are all performed on the mother, and are intended to detect traits or characteristics of a fetus with an abnormality. Once initial screening tests have recognised an increased risk of a potential abnormality, definitive diagnosis can be made by invasive testing.

Single-gene disorders

Several fetal, single-gene disorders can be detected prenatally. Detection of a disorder is achieved using a combination of DNA analysis, biochemical analysis, ultrasound scanning, and other techniques.

Congenital malformations

Prenatal diagnosis is also possible for the detection of several congenital malformations. The techniques used include the combined use of maternal serum markers, and detailed ultrasound scanning.

MATERNAL SERUM MARKERS

Maternal serum screening involves taking a blood sample from the pregnant mother, and analysing it to see if it contains certain 'markers' of fetal abnormality. Maternal serum markers include alpha-fetoprotein (α-FP), human chorionic gonadotrophin (hCG) and unconjugated oestriol (uE3). The levels of these markers are fed into a formula together with the maternal age, and the measurement of fetal nuchal translucency. A computer program then calculates the individual risk for that particular fetus, and can predict Down's syndrome with 70% sensitivity and 95% specificity (*i.e.* there is a 30% false-negative rate and 5% false-positive rate). In some centres, inhibin A has been added as a fourth serum marker, which increases the sensitivity of the test slightly.

Maternal serum screening for open neural tube defects, such as spina bifida, are most accurate when performed at 16–18 weeks' gestation, but generally serum screening tests are carried out at 12 weeks' gestation, as the majority mothers are keen for an early indication of fetal health. If termination of pregnancy would be considered on the basis of a serious abnormality, the sooner the result is known the better.

In the UK, a screening result of 1:250 is considered high-risk, and such a result arises in approximately 5% of pregnancies: these women will be offered amniocentesis or chorionic villus sampling, which provide a far more specific result than serum screening does (see below).

Alpha-fetoprotein

Alpha-fetoprotein is initially made by the yolk sac, and later by the fetal liver. It is present in the fetal blood stream and the amniotic fluid, and some filters through the placenta to reach the maternal blood stream. If the fetus has a neural tube detect, α-FP is elevated as it leaks from the exposed fetal capillaries into the amniotic fluid, and this rise can be detected in the maternal blood. Unexplained elevations of maternal α-FP are associated with an increased risk of spontaneous miscarriage, premature labour, low birth weight and perinatal death.

AMNIOCENTESIS

Amniocentesis is a procedure used in the prenatal diagnosis of genetic abnormalities and fetal infections, in which a small amount of amniotic fluid is extracted from the amniotic sac using needle aspiration. Ultrasound scanning is used to help the clinician direct the needle through the maternal abdomen, uterine wall, through the chorionic cavity and into the amniotic sac (Fig. 3.2). Alternatively, access can be gained through the cervix.

The amniotic fluid contains fetal tissue, from which DNA is extracted and analysed in a laboratory. Amniocentesis can be performed as soon as sufficient amniotic fluid surrounds the fetus, which is usually by 15 weeks' gestation. The most common abnormalities tested for are Down's syndrome, trisomy 18, and spina bifida. The

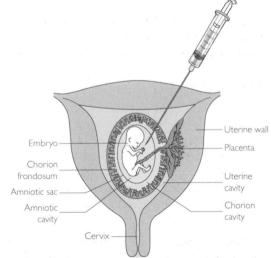

Figure 3.2 The fetus and membranes.

sensitivity of measurement of amniotic fluid α-FP is 100% for anencephaly and > 98% for open spina bifida (but remember these conditions are both visible on ultrasound scanning).

Risks associated with amniocentesis

Amniocentesis carries risks of introducing infection into the amniotic sac and causing trauma to the fetus resulting in limb deformities. Occasionally, there is failure of the needle puncture site to heal properly; this will result in amniotic fluid leakage, and the development of oligohydramnios. Allo-immunisation may also occur in Rhesus-negative mothers who are carrying a Rhesus-positive fetus. To prevent this, all Rhesus-negative mothers are given anti-D antibody at time of amniocentesis. Miscarriage occurs in 0.5% of pregnancies following amniocentesis.

CHORIONIC VILLUS SAMPLING

Chorionic villus sampling involves taking a sample of the chorionic villus and testing it. The sample is harvested by passing a thin needle either through the abdomen, or through the cervix into the chorionic plate under ultrasound guidance.

Advantage of chorionic villus sampling

The advantage of chorionic villous sampling is that it can be carried out earlier than amniocentesis, at 12 weeks' gestation. Sampling done at gestations earlier than this, although possible, results in a high incidence of digital amputation abnormalities and cleft palate.

Risks associated with chorionic villus sampling

Chorionic villus sampling carries a slightly higher risk of miscarriage than amniocentesis, of 1–2%. This is thought to be as the background rate of spontaneous miscarriage at this early gestation and is higher than in the second trimester. Chorionic villus sampling carries similar risks of infection and amniotic fluid leakage as does amniocentesis. Occasionally, maternal cells can contaminate the sample and, because some pregnancies show placental mosaicism, some fetal defects may be missed.

THE 12-WEEK NUCHAL SCAN

The 12-week 'nuchal' scan is often the first ultrasound scan routinely carried out during pregnancy (Fig. 3.3). It is performed in order to: (i) confirm the viability of the fetus; (ii) determine whether the woman is carrying a singleton or multiple pregnancy; (iii) calculate the gestation of the pregnancy; and (iv) help estimate risk of a major fetal abnormality.

In practice, the nuchal scan is carried out at 11–13 weeks' gestation. After 14 weeks' gestation, the fetal lymphatic system is sufficiently developed to drain away excess fluid from the nuchal area, and as such is not useful in screening for fetal abnormality.

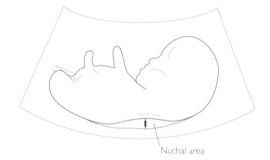

Nuchal area

Figure 3.3 Illustration of ultrasound scan of fetus at 12 weeks' gestation.

The nuchal scan assesses the size of the fluid-filled gap behind the neck of the fetus, to gain a reading described as 'nuchal translucency'. The nuchal scan is performed with the fetus in sagittal section, with the fetal head in neutral position (the fetal neck neither flexed nor extended). The maximum thickness of the nuchal area then is measured. A fetus with Down's syndrome usually has more than the expected amount of fluid present.

THE 20-WEEK ANOMALY SCAN

The anomaly scan is performed between 18–22 weeks' gestation. It is a detailed scan to look at many parts of the fetus, and identify any potential problems. The mother should be made aware that not every abnormality can be picked up on this scan, and that this scan is not a guarantee of normality. Organs examined include:

- **The head:** the skull bones, brain, ventricles, orbits, lips, and ears. Measurements are taken of the biparietal diameter and head circumference. Looks for hydrocephalus.
- **The spine:** each vertebra is visualised, and the overlying skin. Looks for spina bifida.
- **The chest:** the heart and its outflow tracts, the lungs and the diaphragm.
- **The abdomen:** the kidneys, stomach, intestines, bladder, abdominal wall and cord insertion site.
- **The limbs:** the femur length is measured, and this, taken along with the biparietal diameter, is used to estimate gestational age. Possible causes of short femur length are intra-uterine growth restriction (often caused by a chromosomal abnormality), or a skeletal dysplasia.

CHROMOSOMAL ABNORMALITIES

AUTOSOMAL ABNORMALITIES: ANEUPLOIDIES

Aneuploidies is the term given to abnormality of one or more of the autosomal chromosomes. The majority of cases occur due to non-dysjunction in meiosis to cause a trisomy. Non-dysjunction becomes more frequent with increasing maternal age. The vast majority of aneuploidies result in first trimester miscarriage.

Down's syndrome

Down's syndrome is caused by trisomy of chromosome 21. The overall incidence in the UK is 1 in 700 live births. The incidence of Down's syndrome at conception is thought to be much higher, with many conceptions affected by Down's syndrome aborting spontaneously.

The incidence of Down's syndrome increases significantly with increasing maternal age (Table 3.1), but most children with Down's syndrome are born to mothers under the age of 35 years (as there is a higher birth rate in that age group).

Clinical features of Down's syndrome include up-slanting palpebral fissures, a flat occiput, low-set ears, single palmar creases, and wide sandal gaps between first and second toes (Fig. 3.4). Learning disability is common; the intelligence test score (IQ) is usually less than 50, but is very variable. Congenital heart malformations, duodenal atresia, cataracts, epilepsy, hypothyroidism, acute leukaemia, atlanto-axial instability and pre-senile dementia are all common features. The lifespan is rarely longer than 50 years.

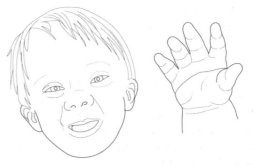

Figure 3.4 Illustrative example of child with Down's syndrome.

Edward's syndrome

Edward's syndrome is caused by trisomy of chromosome 18, the vast majority of cases resulting from maternal non-dysjunction. Of affected fetuses, 95% abort spontaneously. Edward's syndrome is characterised by multiple, characteristic, dysmorphic features (Fig. 3.5). These include small chin, prominent occiput, low-set ears, clenched hands with overlapping index and fifth fingers, single

Table 3.1 Incidence of Down's syndrome with maternal age

Maternal age (years)	Incidence (live births)
20	1:1500
30	1:800
35	1:270
40	1:100
45	1:50

palmar creases, rocker-bottom feet, short sternum, and cryptorchidism (in male babies). Of affected babies, 90% die within the first year of life, and those that survive show profound developmental delay.

Patau's syndrome

Patau's syndrome is caused by trisomy of chromosome 13, again resulting in most cases from maternal non-dysjunction. Neonates with Patau's syndrome have cleft lip and palate (Fig. 3.6), polydactyly and prominent heels. Of affected babies, 90% die within the first year, and those that survive show profound developmental delay.

Triploidy

Triploidy is when, instead of having 46 chromosomes (23 pairs), the fetus has 69 chromosomes (23 groups of 3). This is usually because the egg has been fertilised by two sperms. This is not compatible with life; 99% spontaneously abort, but of those born there is very low birth weight, syndactyly, and hydatidiform-like changes in many cases. Death usually occurs within hours of birth.

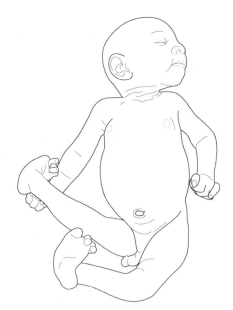

Figure 3.5 Illustrative example of child with Edward's syndrome.

SEX CHROMOSOME ABNORMALITIES

The prevalence of sex chromosome abnormalities does not increase in frequency with increasing maternal age as with aneuploidies.

Turner's syndrome

Turner's syndrome is due to monosomy X (there is only one sex chromosome instead of two), meaning that a female's chromosome complement is 45XO. The incidence is 1 in 5000 female births. Over 99% of affected fetuses spontaneously abort but, once born, life-span is normal. The diagnosis of Turner's syndrome is often only made as a teenager when primary amenorrhoea and short stature begin to be noticed. There is no adolescent growth spurt, a broad chest with widely spaced nipples, webbed neck, a wide carrying angle, and short fourth metacarpals. These females are infertile as they have streak ovaries with no eggs. However, in rare cases, ovarian degeneration is not complete and very occasionally pregnancies can occur.

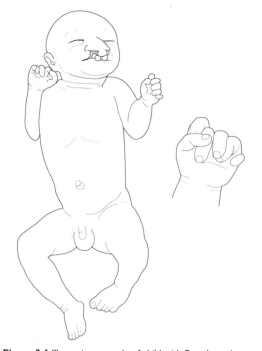

Figure 3.6 Illustrative example of child with Patau's syndrome.

Klinefelter's syndrome

Klinefelter's syndrome is due to XXY karyotype, and occurs in 1 in 1000 male births. Klinefelter's syndrome often goes undetected, only coming to light when investigating subfertility. Klinefelter's syndrome is the single commonest cause of hypogonadism in men. The testes are small and fail to produce adult levels of testosterone. This leads to poorly developed secondary sexual characteristics, and gynaecomastia.

XYY males

Individuals with XYY genotype in essence have an extra male chromosome (Y). XYY males are usually asymptomatic, although intelligence is often lower than average. There is controversial evidence that XYY males are associated with behavioural problems and violent tendencies, with XYY men being over-represented among prison inmates.

HAEMOGLOBINOPATHIES

Sickle cell anaemia

Sickle cell anaemia is an autosomal recessive condition. The disease is characterised by disabling anaemia, painful sickle crises and an increased risk of infections. The carrier prevalence among Africans in some areas is as high as 20%; this is thought to be because the carrier state, that is the heterozygous condition, carries significant selective advantage in making the individual more resistant to malaria.

All pregnant women in the UK of African or Caribbean origin are routinely offered screening to see whether they carry the sickle cell trait. If positive, the partner is offered testing. If both partners carry the sickle cell trait, amniocentesis or chorionic villus sampling is offered in order to determine the fetal genotype.

Long-term complications of sickle cell disease are mainly due to vaso-occlusive events, and include stroke, myocardial infarction, and autosplenectomy. Acute 'sickle chest' is the commonest cause of death, and is caused by infection, fat embolism from necrotic bone marrow, or pulmonary infarction due to sequestration of sickle cells.

Pregnant women with sickle cell disease are managed by obstetricians and haematologists. There should be regular fetal growth assessment by ultrasound, and infection and dehydration should be prevented or promptly treated.

GOOD PRACTICE POINTS 3.8

- Sickle cell anaemia is autosomal recessive. That means if both parents are carriers, there is a 25% chance that each child will have sickle cell disease. If one parent is a carrier, there is a 50% that each child will be a carrier, but none of the children will have the full disease. If one parent has sickle cell disease and the other is a carrier there is a 50% chance that each child will have full sickle cell disease.

BETA-THALASSAEMIA

Beta-thalassaemia is another autosomal recessive condition. It causes malformation of the β-chains of haemoglobin. This results in ineffective erythropoeisis and anaemia to varying degrees:

- Thalassaemia minor (commonly referred to as thalassaemia trait) is asymptomatic.

- Thalassaemia intermedia causes anaemia, with bone deformity, leg ulcers and gallstones, but individuals often manage quite well.

- Thalassaemia major causes a severe anaemia that presents in the first year of life with failure to thrive, recurrent bacterial infections, hepatosplenomegaly and bone expansion. Regular blood transfusions and folic acid are required throughout life.

Alpha-thalassaemia

Alpha-thalassaemia is the result of spontaneous gene deletions that result in malformation or absence of the α-chain of haemoglobin. If one or two genes are absent, the child is asymptomatic. If three genes are absent, infants will have moderate anaemia and splenomegaly, but are able to survive independently. If all four genes are absent, there will be no production of the α-chain of haemoglobin at all. This is incompatible with life, and infants are either still-born at

28–40 weeks' gestation, or are born with a fatal condition known as hydrops fetalis. Such babies are pale and oedematous, with enormous hepatomegaly. They die during the neonatal period.

PRE-EXISTING MEDICAL CONDITIONS THAT AFFECT PREGNANCY

MENTAL HEALTH ISSUES DURING PREGNANCY

Pregnancy is a very emotional time for any woman. Emotional lability is common, and is sometimes explained away as natural, and due to high levels of circulating hormones. Most women, their partners and family cope excellently, and all that is required from the healthcare professional is understanding and re-assurance. However, some feelings can be unhelpful and problematic.

The risk of developing a new mental illness during pregnancy is low, but certainly can happen. For women who suffer from mental illness prior to conception, pregnancy may result in relapse, or worsening of their pre-existing condition; it is important that this is recognised, if it occurs. It is, therefore, important to monitor pregnant women with a personal or family history of mental illness closely within the primary care environment, and to refer them to psychiatric services whenever necessary. Remember that suicide is the second most frequent cause of death amongst pregnant and post-partum women.

Anxiety during pregnancy

Restricting emotions such as anxiety can be intensified during pregnancy, particularly so if there has been a previous pregnancy loss, or if the pregnancy is a result of assisted conception. In such cases, multidisciplinary support from the GP, midwife, obstetrician, and mental health services can be very effective.

Depression during pregnancy

USEFUL WEBSITE

- Depression in pregnancy care: supporting those affected by antenatal depression and anxiety <http://dipcare.org>.

- Depression in pregnancy information leaflet <http://www.patient.co.uk/doctor/Depression-in-Pregnancy.htm>.

The incidence of depression during pregnancy is thought to be far higher than is formally diagnosed, and suicide is a recognised cause of avoidable maternal death. For every 1000 live births, it is estimated that 100–150 women will suffer a depressive illness and 1–2 women will develop a puerperal psychosis. Failure to treat either disorder may result in a prolonged, deleterious effect on the relationship between the mother and her baby. This can have a knock-on effect to the child's psychological, social and educational development. The relationship between a depressed mother and her partner will also be put under strain.

Antenatal depression is one of the strongest predictors for the development of post-natal depression and, in turn, post-natal depression is one of the strongest predictors for the development of parenting stress. It is, therefore, important that antenatal depression is picked up early and treated appropriately. This may require the involvement of perinatal psychiatric services.

Antipsychotic and antidepressant medication during pregnancy

The benefits of continuing antipsychotic or antidepressant medication during pregnancy outweigh the risks to the fetus in most cases. An exception to this is lithium, which is teratogenic if taken in the first trimester; it is, therefore, recommended that women on lithium should come off lithium prior to conception. This will require careful psychiatric monitoring as weaning off lithium can be difficult, and it carries the constant possibility that relapse of the mental illness occurs. Specialist psychiatric input is vital.

THE MOTHER WITH DIABETES MELLITUS

Ideally, every diabetic woman should consult her GP prior to attempting to conceive. This is in order to maximise the likelihood of achieving a good outcome for the pregnancy.

For diabetic women dependent on insulin prior to conception, it is often appropriate that an early referral is made to an obstetrician prior to conception to discuss the risks associated with pregnancy. The obstetrician may mention the following:

- The fetus will carry a higher risk of developing a congenital abnormality and, particularly, of developing a heart defects and/or retinopathy.
- There will be a higher risk of miscarriage and still-birth.
- There will be a higher risk of macrosomia, obstructed labour, and shoulder dystocia.
- There will be a higher risk of pre-eclampsia, eclampsia, keto-acidosis, hypoglycaemia, and infection.

Dietary advice for diabetic mothers

Optimal periconceptual blood glucose control will improve the outlook for both mother and baby; therefore, diabetic control should be optimised for all women prior to conceiving, aiming for an HbA1C < 50 mmol/mol new International Federation of Clinical Chemistry and Laboratory Medicine (IFCC) aligned (this is equivalent to 7% Diabetes Control and Complications Trial [DCCT] aligned). All diabetics should be given an opportunity to discuss their diet with a suitably qualified professional. A dietician, if available, is ideal for this job, but the GP or practice nurse should also be equipped to provide basic guidance.

Folic acid is advised at the higher dose of 5 mg daily.

Metformin

The BNF advises that metformin should be avoided in pregnancy; so once pregnancy has been confirmed, metformin should be stopped. If possible, it is best to control diabetes with dietary restrictions alone; however, should this not be effective, the woman should be started on an insulin regimen.

Insulin

Insulin is safe throughout pregnancy, but insulin requirements will change as the pregnancy progresses, and insulin requirements must be assessed frequently by an experienced physician. This should be in the context of a multidisciplinary antenatal team with a specialist midwife, diabetologist, obstetrician and dietician.

It is usually recommended that labour is induced at 38 weeks of gestation for pregnant diabetic women on insulin. The aim is to achieve a vaginal delivery unless a caesarean section is indicated for other reasons.

THE MOTHER WITH HYPERTENSION

Women who are hypertensive prior to conception carry a higher risk of developing pre-eclampsia during pregnancy than normotensive women. Blood pressure should be optimised prior to attempting to conceive and hypertensive pregnant women require close monitoring of blood pressure and regular checks for proteinuria.

Anti-hypertensive medication

Most anti-hypertensive medications are potentially harmful to the fetus:

- Angiotensin-converting enzyme (ACE) inhibitors may adversely affect fetal renal function and cause skull defects.
- Beta-blockers may cause intra-uterine growth restriction and neonatal bradycardia.
- Calcium channel blockers are not known to cause harm, but manufacturers advise avoidance.

The preferred anti-hypertensive agent for use during pregnancy is methyl-dopa, which is usually administered as a three times daily regimen. In complicated hypertensive patients, care should be managed by a hypertensive specialist.

THE MOTHER WITH A THROMBOTIC DISORDER

There are a number of different thrombotic disorders, any of which can affect a woman of child-bearing age. These include anti-phospholipid syndrome, protein C or protein S deficiency, antithrombin deficiency, Factor V Leiden and many more. Most of these thrombotic disorders are genetic diseases which follow autosomal dominant inheritance.

Pregnancy complications due to thrombotic disorders

Thrombotic disorders can cause recurrent early miscarriages, an increased risk of placental abruption, intra-uterine growth restriction and intra-uterine death. Any woman who has experienced three or more consecutive miscarriages should be tested for a thrombotic disorder.

Management of thrombotic disorders in pregnancy

Haematology is a specialist area and so it is recommended that a pregnant woman carrying a thrombotic disorder should be managed by joint care between the GP and Haematology. Women with a proven thrombophilia will need to take aspirin 75 mg daily before conception, and to continue this throughout pregnancy.

THE MOTHER WITH EPILEPSY

Epilepsy is a chronic disorder that affects approximately 1% of the UK population. It is characterised by unpredictable, paroxysmal seizures which may be focal or generalised. Epilepsy may have an underlying cause, such as brain injury or chronic substance abuse, but more often is idiopathic. Sometimes, epilepsy runs in families, and there is increasing evidence that it does have a genetic component. Epilepsy can be severely debilitating, especially if poorly controlled, and is a particular problem for the pregnant woman as seizures put her at increased risk of falls, during which she may sustain trauma to both herself and the fetus.

Pregnancy complications due to epilepsy

There is an increased risk of congenital abnormality in babies of epileptic mothers. The fetus is fairly resistant to hypoxia during seizures; however, if the woman goes into status epilepticus (a state of uncontrolled seizure lasting over 30 minutes), this will be dangerous for both mother and baby. About 30% of epileptic women have an increase in seizure frequency during pregnancy. This is possibly due to poor compliance with anticonvulsants during pregnancy.

Management of epilepsy during pregnancy

Due to the complexity of epilepsy, the many different types of epilepsy, and individual variability, all epileptic women should be managed by a neurologist, and it is particularly important that she attends her appointments during pregnancy.

Anti-convulsant therapy during pregnancy

The clear benefits of taking anti-convulsants during pregnancy usually outweigh the risks; as a general rule, it is usually recommended that an epileptic trying to conceive should continue on her current anticonvulsant medication. This decision is often difficult to make, and advice from the neurologist, obstetrician, GP, as well as individual patient preference and life-style must all be taken into account.

It is recommended that all pregnant women taking anticonvulsants should take the dietary supplement folic acid at the higher dose of 5 mg daily throughout the pregnancy and vitamin K 10 mg daily from 36 weeks' gestation onwards.

Pregnant epileptics should be scanned by a fetal medicine specialist because of the increased risk of fetal abnormality. All the commonly prescribed anticonvulsants cross the placenta and are teratogenic. There is an association between sodium valproate and neural tube defects. Other major malformations linked to anticonvulsants are cleft lip and palate and congenital heart defects.

Any individual who suffers from epilepsy must not drive a car unless fit free for at least one year. The DVLA should be made aware of the condition.

SPECIAL ANTENATAL AREAS

MULTIPLE PREGNANCY

Multiple pregnancies are usually discovered at the routine 12-week ultrasound scan, but may be suspected at an earlier stage, particularly if there is significant hyperemesis gravidarium, a family history of twins, or conception was a result of fertility treatment. An early scan allows chorionicity to be determined.

Complications of multiple pregnancy

Complications of twin and higher multiple pregnancies are many and are more likely to affect monochorionic pregnancies. Complications affecting the fetuses include fetal malformation, twin-to-twin transfusion syndrome, prematurity, intra-uterine growth restriction, malpresentation, placenta praevia, and intra-uterine death.

Complications affecting the mother include anaemia, gestational diabetes, hypertension, and a higher risk of thrombo-embolism. Therefore, all twin and higher multiple pregnancies, once confirmed by ultrasound scanning, are automatically referred to an obstetrician for close monitoring.

TEENAGE PREGNANCY

The UK has the highest rate of teenage conceptions, abortions and birth rates in Western Europe, with over 40,000 under 18-year-olds becoming pregnant each year. Over 7,000 of these are aged under 16 years. Teenage pregnancy is associated with low socio-economic status, poor educational achievement, and single-parent families, and the great majority of teenage mothers become wholly reliant on social benefits and council housing following delivery.

Many teenage pregnancies are not planned, and many young mothers are shocked to find themselves pregnant, even when they had not been using contraception. However, it should not be forgotten that some teenage pregnancies are planned and wanted.

Teenage pregnancy strategy

The teenage pregnancy strategy is attempting to lower the high teenage conception rate in the UK, and is showing some success in some areas, by providing education in schools and the media regarding sex and relationships, and by increasing access for young people to contraceptive services. The strategy also attempts to provide support to teenage mothers to help them gain some form of education or employment after the birth.

OLDER MOTHERHOOD

In the UK, there has been an almost 50% increase in the number of women over the age of 40 years having giving birth in the last 10 years. There has also been an increase in the number of women over the age of 50 years giving birth. In 2006, there were 71 such births in the UK.

Complications associated with older motherhood

Increasing age carries a higher risk of the fetus having Down's syndrome and other chromosomal abnormalities.

Older motherhood also carries a higher risk of non-pregnancy-related complications such as ischaemic heart disease and stroke, as well as pregnancy-related complications such as varicose veins, sciatica, hyperemesis and fatigue. There is also some evidence that perinatal morbidity rates increase after 40 weeks' gestation in mothers over the age of 40 years, who may, therefore, be offered elective induction at term. Despite this, older mothers are often more financially secure, more often in a stable supportive relationship, are more experienced in life, and are consequently in many ways more fit than younger women to cope with the strains of pregnancy.

Older pregnant women are treated the same way as any other woman during her pregnancy. Any problems or complications (of which there may be none) are managed as they arise.

SUBSTANCE MISUSE DURING PREGNANCY

Cocaine

Cocaine carries a risk of early miscarriage, intra-uterine growth restriction, low birth weight, neonatal cerebral infarction, congenital abnormality, placental abruption, and still-birth.

Opiates

Opiates carry the risk of early miscarriage, multiple gestation, intra-uterine growth restriction, low birth weight, preterm labour, and neonatal opiate withdrawal syndrome.

Cannabis

Cannabis carries a risk of preterm labour.

Alcohol

Alcohol carries a risk of fetal alcohol syndrome, intra-uterine growth restriction, and low birth weight. Alcohol can also lead to maternal malnutrition. Vitamin B and iron supplements are, therefore, advised for pregnant women with a high alcohol intake, and advice should be in order to promote a healthy eating habit.

Tobacco

Smoking carries risk of intra-uterine growth restriction, low birth weight, antepartum haemorrhage, increased overall perinatal mortality, and leukaemia in childhood. Interestingly, smoking decreases the risk of developing pre-eclampsia.

IMMIGRATION ISSUES FOR PREGNANT WOMEN

Many women who are not British citizens deliver their babies in the UK. They may be professionals working here or spouses of such, refugees with leave to remain, asylum seekers, illegal immigrants, foreign students or simply tourists in the UK on holiday.

All women, no matter what their ethnic origin or status, currently have the legal right to receive primary care and emergency care free at the point of need. If labour begins while in the UK, emergency care would constitute full support during labour including ambulance transport to hospital, analgesia, midwife assistance, and surgical obstetric assistance, as required.

It is suspected that some women travel to the UK to deliver their babies on the National Health Service, and thus receive good quality care during labour, free of charge. This, however, is against National Health Service regulations, and women may be issued a fee on discharge. This is currently a hot topic of both ethical and political debate.

MATERNAL MORTALITY

The maternal mortality rate is the number of deaths per 100,000 pregnant women. It includes women who die during pregnancy and within 42 days of delivery, miscarriage or abortion.

DIRECT DEATHS

Direct deaths are defined as those related to obstetric complications or any treatment received during pregnancy, labour or puerperium (the 6 weeks' post-partum). The direct death rate in the UK is currently 5.3 per 100,000 women. Causes of direct deaths in the UK include pulmonary embolus, haemorrhage, eclampsia, ectopic pregnancy and sepsis.

INDIRECT DEATHS

Indirect deaths are those associated with a pre-existing disorder, the effect of which is exacerbated by pregnancy or an irrelevant cause such as a road traffic accident. The indirect death rate in the UK is currently 7.8 per 100,000 women. These figures show that one woman in 7600 will die due to pregnancy in the UK. This is contrasted with one woman in seven who will die due to pregnancy in Niger.

RISK FACTORS FOR MATERNAL DEATH

There are some clear indicators that identify women in the UK who are more likely to succumb to a maternal death.

Social disadvantage

The maternal mortality rate is 20 times higher in the unemployed and socially excluded section of society when compared to the highest social classes. The maternal mortality rate is three times higher in single mothers compared to those women with a supportive partner.

Minority ethnic groups

The maternal mortality rate is three times higher in women from minority ethnic groups when compared with Caucasian women. Asylum seekers and newly arrived refugees have a maternal mortality rate seven times higher than that of British Caucasian women.

Late booking or poor attendance

One-fifth of women who die in pregnancy book in for their antenatal care after 22 weeks' gestation, or miss over four antenatal visits.

Obesity

One-third of women who die in pregnancy are clinically obese.

FETAL AND NEONATAL MORTALITY

STILL-BIRTH

Still-birth is delivery of a dead fetus that has a gestational age of at least 24 weeks. The baby shows no sign of life, and the Apgar score at 1 and 5 minutes is 0.

Still-birth may be expected, such as following a known intra-uterine death and induction of labour, or unexpected, following what had started off as a normal labour. Whether expected or not, it is a very distressing moment for the mother and all involved. If it is known that death has occurred *in utero*, the delivery is usually carried out in a specially designated room, by a midwife experienced in caring for perinatal loss cases.

Management of still-births

The mother should be allowed time with her baby, even if such is in poor condition, as this has been shown to help the grieving process. The mortuary technician may provide suitably sized cots and clothes in which to dress the baby, and some will take foot and handprints if the parents would like this as a memento.

Cabergoline 1 g stat can be given to the mother in order to suppress lactation, as breasts heavy with milk can be rather distressing when there is no baby to feed.

Examination of still-born babies

A post mortem examination may be helpful to confirm the presence of suspected fetal abnormalities or to rule them out. Some parents are horrified at the thought of their baby undergoing post mortem whereas others welcome the chance to gain as much information as possible about why their baby died. Whether or not to allow a post mortem examination on their baby is a difficult decision for parents, and the pros and cons must be explained sensitively by a senior obstetrician when deciding whether to opt for post-mortem examination or not. The birthing assistant present at the delivery (usually the midwife) should document details of the baby's external appearance, in case this is the only 'examination' carried out. Following post mortem, the body will be released for burial or cremation. Disposal of a late miscarriage is a sensitive subject, and care should be taken to ascertain the mother's wishes.

Registration of still-birth

All still-births must be registered at the hospital or local registry office within 42 days of the still-birth. In order to do this, a medical certificate of still-birth must be issued by the doctor or midwife who was present at the time of delivery. All stillbirths are then reported to CEMACH, the Confidential Enquiry into Maternal and Child Health.

NEONATAL DEATH

> ### Useful Website
>
> - Foundation for Study of Infant Deaths <www.fsid.org.uk>.
>
> - SANDS, the Stillbirth and Neonatal Death Society <www.uk-sands.org>.

Neonatal death is the term given when a baby is born alive, at over 24 weeks' gestation, but dies within 7 days of delivery. If a baby is born before 24 weeks' gestation, it is termed a miscarriage if it showed no signs of life. If the baby showed signs of life and then died, it is classified as a neonatal death, even if it was born before 24 weeks' gestation.

Perinatal mortality rate

Perinatal mortality rate (PMR) is the number of still-births plus the number of early neonatal deaths per 1000 deliveries. In the UK, the PMR rate is 8 per 1000 deliveries.

Cot death

Cot death is the sudden and unexpected death of a baby for no apparent reason. Approximately 300 babies die of cot death each year in the UK. Cot death is sometimes referred to as sudden infant death syndrome (SIDS). The majority of cot deaths occur before the age of 1 year. Babies should always be placed on their back to sleep, in order to reduce the risk of cot death.

Follow-up for women who have experienced still-birth or neonatal death

Women should be offered an appointment with an obstetrician following the still-birth or neonatal death to discuss whether anything went wrong and to receive advice regarding possible future pregnancies. Many hospitals also provide a women's health counsellor who may even do home visits.

Module 4:
Management of labour and delivery

You will be expected to have the knowledge, understanding and judgement to be capable of initial management of intrapartum problems in a hospital and in a community setting. This will include: knowledge and understanding of normal and abnormal labour, data and investigation interpretation, induction and augmentation of labour, assessment of fetal well-being and compromise.

An understanding of the management of all obstetric emergencies is expected.

You will need to demonstrate appropriate knowledge of regional anaesthesia, analgesia and operative delivery including caesarean section.

You will need to be able to demonstrate respect for cultural and religious differences in attitudes to childbirth.

odule four concerns delivery of the fetus and the transition of the pregnant woman into motherhood. The normal vaginal delivery is explained, and there are ample diagrams provided to help visualise this process. Difficult and obstructed labours are explained in a way that an obstetric specialist trainee would be able to manage emergencies, and a GP would be able to conduct a home delivery safely. It is also important for GPs to have a secure grasp of the activities of the labour ward, as often questions arise from new mothers only once things have settled down, and she is back at home.

USEFUL WEBSITE

- NICE Guidance: Intrapartum care: management and delivery of care to women in labour <http://guidance.nice.org.uk/CG55>.

NORMAL LABOUR

Labour is the process by which the fetus, placenta and membranes are expelled from the uterus, through the birth canal into the outside world. Labour is the natural culmination of approximately 40 weeks of pregnancy, and results in new life being born.

Normal labour occurs when it starts spontaneously at term (37–42 weeks' gestation), the fetus presents by the vertex, and is delivered without complication, or the need for any medical intervention.

THE WEEKS PRIOR TO DELIVERY

During the 3 weeks prior to labour, certain changes occur which indicate that the onset of labour is soon approaching.

Engagement of the fetal head

The pelvic brim is the imaginary boundary of the entrance (superior part) of the pelvis. When more than 60% of the fetal head has sunk past the pelvic brim into the pelvis, the fetus is said to be engaged. This can be assessed by palpation.

In primagravid women and those with strong abdominal wall muscles, the fundal height will sink only slightly. In multiparous women and those with weak abdominal wall muscles, the fetal head may not engage and the fetus becomes pendulous within the abdomen, making walking difficult. Back pain can be a problem, as can urinary frequency which occurs due to pressure of the fetal head on the maternal urinary bladder. The laxity of the pelvic floor muscles sometimes results in urinary incontinence.

Braxton Hicks contractions

Braxton Hicks contractions, which will have been felt from about 20 weeks, may be felt more often as the onset of labour approaches. These are non-painful uterine contractions that last 1–2 minutes.

GOOD PRACTICE POINT 4.1

- Remember Braxton Hicks contractions are not painful.

CERVICAL SHORTENING

The cervix shortens and becomes merged with the lower uterine segment.

ONSET OF LABOUR

It is unclear what exactly precipitates the onset of normal labour, but it is likely to be a combination of a number of factors, both maternal and fetal. Distension of the uterus and pressure of the fetal head on the cervix is the likely to be the main precipitant of labour. It is possible that the feto–placental unit provides some signal that it is ready to move and be delivered, but this signal has not been elucidated as yet. Progesterone, the main hormone support of pregnancy, drops, and oxytocin, a uterine stimulant, starts to be released from the posterior pituitary gland to enhance uterine contractions.

Onset of true labour

The onset of true labour is recognised by regular, painful, uterine contractions. Labour is divided into three stages for the convenience of healthcare workers:

> *Stage 1* – from onset of true labour to full dilation of the cervix.
>
> *Stage 2* – from full cervical dilation to expulsion of the fetus.
>
> *Stage 3* – From birth of the baby to expulsion of the placenta and membranes.

THE FIRST STAGE

Duration of labour

Duration of labour varies greatly with parity. The total duration of labour is approximately 12 hours for a primiparous woman, and 7 hours for a parous woman. It is the first stage which takes most of the time; dilatation of the cervix takes on average 1 hour to dilate 1 cm in primiparous women, and 30 minutes to dilate 1 cm in parous women.

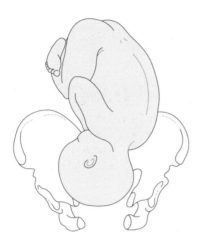

Figure 4.1 Descent of fetus in left occipito-anterior position.

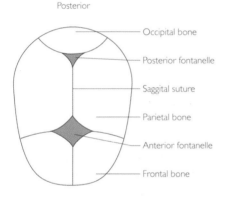

Posterior

— Occipital bone

— Posterior fontanelle

— Saggital suture

— Parietal bone

— Anterior fontanelle

— Frontal bone

Anterior

Figure 4.2 Fetal skull (seen from above).

Descent of the fetus

Descent of the fetal head may occur 2–3 weeks prior to the onset of labour, resulting in most of the fetal head sinking below the pelvic brim for the start of labour. The regular, strong, painful, uterine contractions that characterise the onset of labour force the fetus to descend further into the pelvis so that the full fetal head passes the pelvic brim. At this time, the body of the fetus usually lies slightly to the left (less often to the right), and the face usually looks toward the mother's right ilium. If the fetal spine lies to the left, this would be known as left occipito-anterior position (Fig. 4.1).

The position of the head can be identified by vaginal examination by feeling for the anterior fontanelle, and the sagittal suture (Fig. 4.2).

Flexion of the fetal neck

As the fetal head descends into the true pelvis, it meets resistance at the pelvic floor. Pressure from the contracting uterus causes the head to flex on the neck (Fig. 4.3).

Internal rotation

The pelvic inlet is not round, but more of an oval shape. Neither is the fetal head or the fetal body round, but both are also an oval shape. This means that the longest part of the head (the occipo-anterior or saggital plane) needs to be aligned with the widest part of the pelvic inlet (the lateral, or coronal plane) in order to fit through. The head does this by passing through the pelvic brim, 'looking to one side', usually looking to the right. Once the fetal head has passed through the inlet, it finds that the pelvis is now long in the saggital plane, and so needs to rotate once again in order to pass through. The fetal body, however, needs to remain

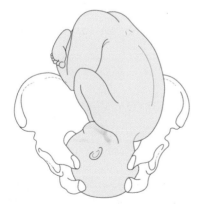

Figure 4.3 Flexion of neck

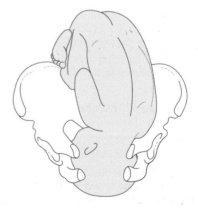

Figure 4.4 Internal rotation.

aligned in the coronal plane for it to pass through the pelvic brim. Therefore, the fetal head rotates on the neck, and is guided to do so by the gutter shape of the pelvic floor and the incessant pushing by the uterus above (Fig. 4.4). The fetus now faces towards the mother's sacrum.

Crowning of the head

Once the occipital prominence escapes under the symphysis pubis, the head no longer recedes between each uterine contraction. This is known as crowning of the head (Fig. 4.5).

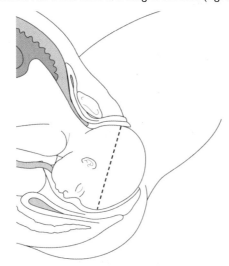

Figure 4.5 Crowning of the fetal head.

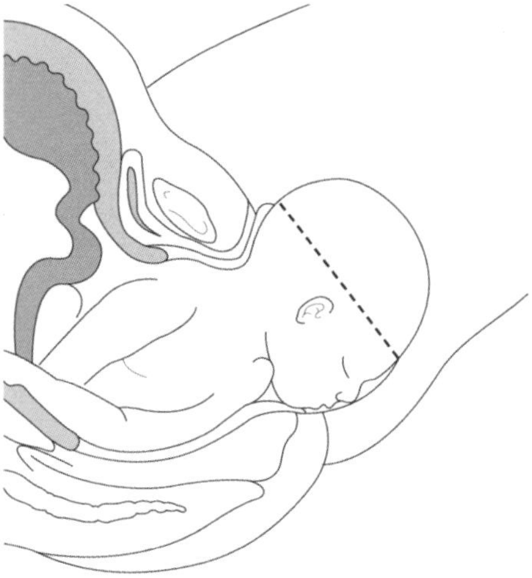

Figure 4.6 Extension of the fetal head.

Extension of the fetal head

The fetal head then extends on the neck and the face sweeps the perineum, and usually looks to the mother's anus (Fig. 4.6).

Restitution

The body of the fetus in the birth canal is still lying slightly on the side (usually the spine lies to the left); however, due to internal rotation of the fetal head on the body, the head comes out aligned anterior–posteriorly, i.e. the fetal head is twisted on the body, and is most probably uncomfortable. The head, once out of the birth canal, therefore re-aligns itself with its body. This is called restitution, and usually results in the baby looking to the mother's right buttock (Fig. 4.7).

Internal rotation of shoulders

Just as the head needed to twist itself so that its longest diameter would be aligned with the longest plane of the pelvic outlet, so does the body. This is known as internal rotation of the shoulders, and usually involves the shoulders and chest turning to face the right, and the buttocks turning to the left (Fig. 4.8).

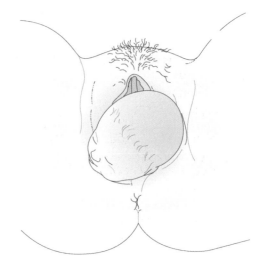

Figure 4.7 Restitution (baby looks at mother's buttock).

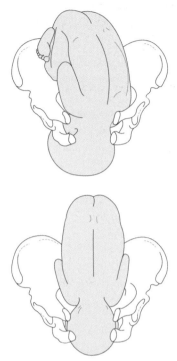

Figure 4.8 Internal rotation of fetal shoulders

Lateral flexion of body

The body of the fetus is then expelled from the birth canal, flexing laterally as the anterior shoulder pivots past the symphysis pubis (Fig. 4.9). The baby is born.

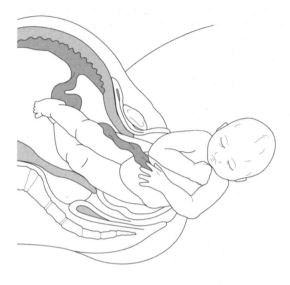

Figure 4.9 Lateral flexion of fetal body.

MANAGEMENT OF NORMAL LABOUR

Normal labour needs to be managed safely and non-intrusively as much as possible. It is important that the mother is examined at regular intervals to ensure that labour is progressing as it should. The partogram is essential as a way of recording the progression of labour, and these partograms are usually filled in by midwives.

The partogram

The partogram (Fig. 4.10 see next page) is a graphical description of the progression of labour. It records the following against time, and plots them on a graph for easy visual interpretation:

- Cervical dilatation.
- Descent of the fetal head.
- Fetal heart rate.
- Uterine contractions (strength and frequency).

Onto the partogram is also recorded maternal blood pressure, temperature and pulse, as well her state of mind. All drugs administered are also noted down.

Perineal tears

Spontaneous perineal and vaginal tears are common during normal vaginal delivery, they are usually small, and heal well.

- First degree tears involve injury to the vaginal epithelium and vulval skin only. They are usually left to heal by themselves.
- Second degree tears involve injury to the perineal muscles. They are usually sutured closed by the midwife soon after delivery.

- Third degree tears involve injury to the anal sphincter. They are usually repaired by the obstetrician in theatre.
- Fourth degree tears involve injury to the rectal mucosa. They are repaired by the obstetrician in theatre, and may require assistance from a colorectal surgeon.

The perineum should be kept clean and dry while it is healing. Many women find ice-packs and simple analgesia helpful. Some obstetric units have a perineal clinic to follow-up women who suffered perineal trauma during child-birth.

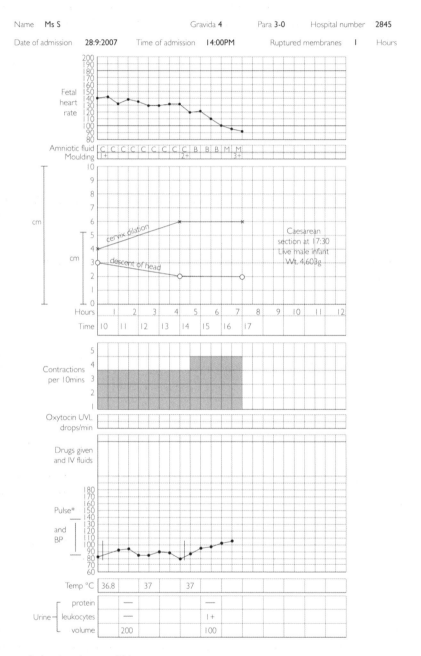

Figure 4.10 Partograph showing obstructed labour.

FIRST-LINE PAIN RELIEF IN LABOUR

By definition, labour is painful; there must be regular, painful, uterine contractions before it is said to have started. Dilatation of the cervix is also painful, particularly in primiparous women. There is a large difference between the levels of pain that women can tolerate; many go through labour successfully without analgesia, particularly in the developing world. However, many women suffer excruciating pain which leaves a mental scar for life. Obstructed labour, primagravid labours, and women with psychological issues suffer from the most pain. Optimistic, well-prepared and socially supported women report the least pain.

There are a number of ways in which the pain of labour can be managed effectively, to make the experience of childbirth tolerable, and even pleasurable.

GOOD PRACTICE POINT 4.2

- Always discuss pain relief choices with women during pregnancy, before they go into labour, to allow them to make an informed choice and maintain a feeling of control when it comes to delivery and decision-making.

Relaxing surroundings

Simple things like having one's own room, not hearing the lady next door screaming, having soft background music and subtle lighting, all help the labouring woman relax and take control of her pain. These details should not be underestimated.

Complementary medicine

Whether homeopathy, acupuncture, and hypnosis work by placebo or otherwise, many women do find these methods immensely beneficial.

TENS machines

Transcutaneous electrical nerve stimulation (TENS) machines are becoming increasingly popular and can be bought quite easily over the counter, on the internet, and are available on some NHS labour wards. TENS machines pass low levels of electric current through the skin via electrodes which are usually placed over L1 and S2 dermatomes. The labouring woman is able to control the frequency of stimulation with a hand-held control. TENS is thought to work by blocking pain stimuli passing through the spinal neuronal gate, and by encouraging endorphin production.

Simple oral analgesis

This includes taking drugs such as paracetamol, ibuprofen, or co-codamol.

'Gas-and-air' (Entonox)

Most women in the UK are familiar with 'gas-and-air' and it is offered first-line to all labouring women. It is available in ambulances. This 'gas-and-air', known as Entonox, is a 50:50 mix of nitrous oxide (laughing gas) and oxygen. It is relatively insoluble in blood and, as such, takes approximately 45 seconds, or six deep breaths, to have its full analgesic effect. Therefore, the labouring woman is instructed to start inhalation as the contraction begins, and stop the inhalation as soon as the pain of contraction starts to ease. It wears off rapidly, so that the labouring woman remains in control and alert throughout. Many women in the UK manage labour well using 'gas and air' alone.

INJECTABLE ANALGESIA

Pethidine

Intramuscular opioid injections provide good, instant, pain relief, and are popular; the drug most commonly used is pethidine 100 mg. Side effects include drowsiness, disorientation, nausea, vomiting and constipation. An anti-emetic such as prochlor-perizine or cyclizine can be given with the pethidine to counter the nausea. Some women express a feeling of loss of control. Opioids are able to cross through the placenta to the fetus; when high doses are used, the neonate may show signs of drowsiness or even opioid overdose after delivery. In rare cases, the baby may require naloxone (an opiate antagonist).

Pudendal nerve injection

The pudendal nerve supplies the vulva and perineum. The nerve can be accessed through the vaginal wall and injected with local anaesthetic. This is useful to assist forceps delivery, but is becoming less commonly used in the UK.

EPIDURAL ANALGESIA

Epidural analgesia involves insertion of a catheter into the extradural space, through which a continuous infusion of local anaesthetic is provided. The extradural space is the area inside the bony spinal canal but outside the dura mater of the spinal cord. It is also known as the epidural space (Fig 4.11). Lignocaine in crystalloid fluid can be used for a short-acting effect, and bupivacaine in crystalloid fluid can be used for a more long-lasting effect. Lumbar epidural analgesia is popular among women for pain control during labour, and can usually be performed on request by the hospital anaesthetic team. Epidural analgesia is generally not available to women delivering at home or in midwife-led birthing units.

Lumbar epidural analgesia provides extremely effective relief from labour pain, so much so that women may be unaware of when they are having uterine contractions, and must rely on a midwife palpating their uterus to inform them of when contractions are occurring, so that they know when to push.

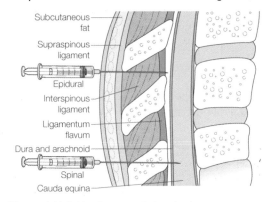

Figure 4.11 Epidural versus spinal analgesia.

Benefits of epidural analgesia

One of the great benefits of epidural analgesia is that, once the epidural catheter has been inserted, it can be easily topped up for long labours and for caesarean section. Epidural analgesia is, therefore, often encouraged if caesarean section seems likely, for example, in vaginal trial after previous caesarean section or in multiple pregnancies. Another benefit of epidural analgesia is that it has a hypotensive effect which can be put into therapeutic use to control pre-eclamptic hypertension.

Drawbacks of epidural analgesia

One of the main drawbacks of epidural analgesia is that, once in place, sometimes the woman can feel confined to her bed; although efforts are made to encourage her to walk around the room with the epidural tubes supported on a mobile stand, this does not always occur. However, although mobilising with an epidural in place requires more effort by the labouring woman and her midwife, it certainly is possible.

The other drawback of concern is that there is an increased rate of assisted delivery when epidural analgesia has been used. This is likely due to a combination of reasons, such as the relaxed pelvic floor not adequately flexing the fetal head during descent, and the mother not feeling the urge to push. Perhaps those women who ask for epidural analgesia would be more likely to have assisted delivery anyway, since they may have longer, and more painful, labours. The evidence is unclear.

There is no substantiation that women who use epidural analgesia during labour experience more chronic back pain post-natally than women who use other methods of pain control. However, it is common for women who experience back pain post-natally to blame the epidural as the cause of their problem.

SPINAL ANALGESIA

Spinal analgesia involves a single injection of local anaesthetic into the subarachnoid space. It produces very effective pain relief which lasts for 2–4 hours. It is quick to perform, and often chosen for caesarean section deliveries or instrumental deliveries.

GENERAL ANAESTHESIA

General anaesthesia is reserved for use only with caesarean section deliveries. It carries risks to both the mother and fetus; the rate of maternal deaths due to general anaesthesia is at least double the rate of deaths due to regional anaesthesia. The primary cause of maternal death due to general anaesthesia is a result of difficulty with airway management; aspiration of gastric contents can result in severe pneumonitis. The greatest risk is a result of decreased uterine blood flow and can result in severe neonatal respiratory depression. It is extremely important that there is senior support for the obstetric anaesthetist when a general anaesthetic has to be administered.

ASSESSMENT OF FETAL WELL-BEING AND COMPROMISE: HOME BIRTH

The National Institute for Health and Clinical Excellence (NICE) guidance on intrapartum care states that all women with uncomplicated pregnancies should be given the option to deliver their baby at home. The Department of Health has pledged to implement this, but there are difficulties in being able to provide enough midwives for this service. Each labouring woman must have one-to-one support from a trained midwife if her delivery is to be safe.

BENEFITS OF HOME BIRTH

There are many clear benefits to home birth. The woman may be more relaxed and comfortable in her own surroundings, and is more likely to remain mobile. Deliveries at home 'demedicalise' what is essentially a natural process, and there is the potential to involve more family members than is possible in hospital, including children (most labour wards only allow one birthing partner to be present during delivery). Women can feel much more in control over their bodies; not having to depend on science, technology, institutions and machines to deliver her baby into the world can give her confidence in knowing that she is the best one to look after her baby in the weeks and months to come. This impression of control can have a long-lasting effect on women, and how they view themselves as a 'good' and 'competent', and must not be disregarded.

Statistics show that deliveries taking place at home are more likely to be achieved without the need for clinical intervention. However, one-fifth of women who intend to deliver at home, develop an unforeseen complication and require transfer to the hospital for assistance. This might be because of poor progress in labour, meconium stained liquor, post partum haemorrhage or neonatal asphyxia. Women considering a home birth must be informed that, should something go unexpectedly seriously wrong in labour, the consequences can be worse than if the complication were to occur in an obstetric unit.

WATER BIRTH

Many women have found comfort lying in a warm bath during their labour. Some women use the birthing pool intermittently, going in and out of the bath as it suits them; others remain in the water throughout labour, and deliver the child underwater. This can be difficult for midwives and requires a lot of effort and experience in water deliveries. However, the results can be encouraging: warm water can have a wonderfully soothing effect on the labouring women and may even mitigate the need for analgesia.

PINARD STETHOSCOPE

All experienced, well-trained midwives and obstetricians will be able to use the Pinard stethoscope to auscultate the fetal heart (Fig. 4.12). The Pinard stethoscope is usually used intermittently and has a number of benefits: it is non-invasive, cheap, light, does not require batteries (important in developing countries) and, most importantly, it is effective. It is not painful or restricting for the mother.

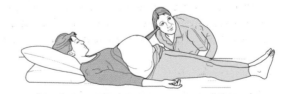

Figure 4.12 Midwife using the Pinard stethoscope.

The fetal heart should be auscultated for a full 60 seconds to make an accurate assessment of fetal well-being. Fetal tachycardia, bradycardia, and late decelerations may all be signs of fetal distress. If such signs are present, cardiotocograph (CTG) monitoring is advisable.

It is reasonable to use the Pinard stethoscope to listen to the fetal heart approximately every 15 minutes during the first stage of labour and after each contraction during the second stage of labour.

The fetal heart rate can also be heard using a hand-held Doppler. This method is very popular with mothers as it allows them to hear their baby's heartbeat themselves, and thus share in the experience.

CARDIOTOCOGRAPH

A cardiotocograph (CTG) is a printed record of the fetal heart rate and maternal uterine contractions. The record of contractions is achieved by strapping a pressure monitor, the tocodynamometer, onto the mother's abdomen using an elastic belt. This may be uncomfortable for the woman and is certainly restrictive. Alternatively, a pressure catheter can be inserted into the uterine cavity; as this requires a degree of cervical dilatation, it is used very infrequently.

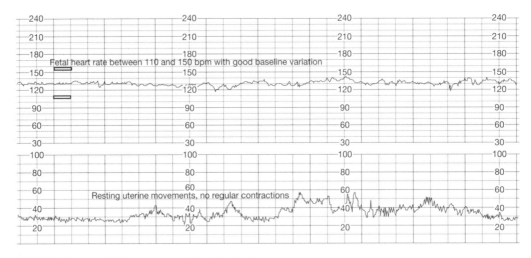

Figure 4.13 Cardiotocograph showing a normal baseline fetal heart rate.

The fetal heart rate can be measured using either a Doppler ultrasound probe strapped to the mother's abdomen above the fetal heart or by the use of a fetal scalp electrode. The fetal scalp electrode is the preferred method only when external abdominal monitoring is unsatisfactory, or for multiple pregnancies where it provides a way of accurately monitoring each twin separately as the fetal scalp electrode effectively avoids the mistake of monitoring the same twin twice and ignoring the other, as can occur with the ultrasound probe. A degree of cervical dilatation, and rupture of the amniotic membranes are required in order to place a fetal scalp electrode on the fetal scalp.

Features of a normal CTG
When a fetus is comfortable, the CTG is quite characteristic:
- *Rate:* a normal baseline fetal heart rate is between 110–150 bpm (Fig. 4.13). Note that the baseline fetal heart rate slows physiologically with advancing gestation.
- *Variability:* the normal variability in the baseline fetal heart rate is between 10–25 bpm.
- *Accelerations:* accelerations of the fetal heart rate with contractions are a sign of a healthy fetus, but their absence in advanced labour is not unusual. Antenatally, there should be at least two accelerations with amplitude of more than 15 bpm, every 15 minutes (Fig. 4.14). Each acceleration should last at least 15 seconds.

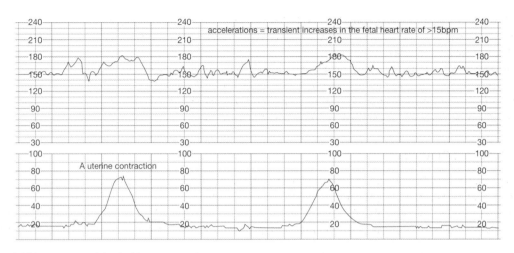

Figure 4.14 Acceleration of the fetal heart rate with contractions.

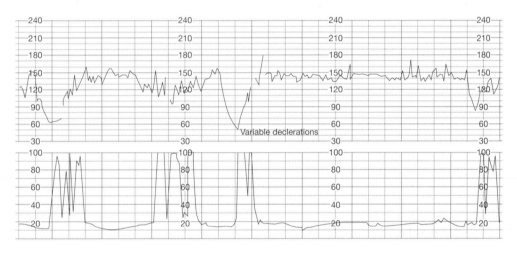

Figure 4.15 Variable decelerations in the fetal heart rate.

Decelerations

'Early decelerations' are transient falls in the fetal heart rate during a uterine contraction. They are normal and likely to represent physiological increased fetal vagal tone due to head compression.

'Variable decelerations' are transient falls in the fetal heart rate that vary in both shape and time. They do not necessarily occur simultaneously with uterine contractions (Fig 4.15). Variable decelerations may be perfectly normal, but may be a sign of compression of the umbilical cord. Changing the mother's position may cause the variable decelerations to cease. A small acceleration at the beginning and end of a deceleration is known as shouldering. This suggests that the fetus is coping well with the stress of the intermittent compressions.

Features of an abnormal CTG

When the fetus is distressed, the CTG changes in well-recognised ways.

- *Baseline rate*: a sustained baseline fetal heart rate of over 150 bpm (tachycardia) or under 110 bpm (bradycardia) is abnormal (Fig. 4.16). Fetal tachycardia may be due to maternal pyrexia, fetal acidosis, or prematurity.

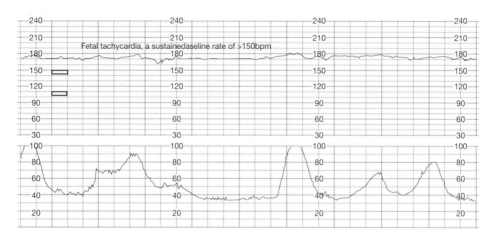

Figure 4.16 Fetal tachycardia.

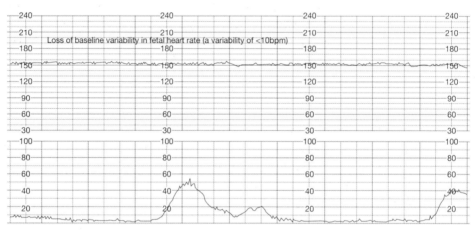

Figure 4.17 Loss of baseline variability in the fetal heart rate.

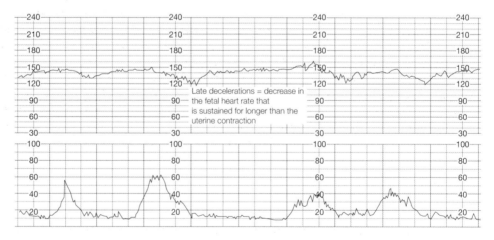

Figure 4.18 Late decelerations in the fetal heart rate after a uterine contraction has relaxed.

- *Loss of baseline variability*: loss of baseline variability (Fig. 4.17) may occur physiologically for up to 40 minutes while the fetus 'sleeps'. Loss of variability is also associated with preterm labour, fetal acidosis, and administration of opioid drugs to the mother.

- *Late decelerations*: a late deceleration is a fall in the fetal heart rate after a uterine contraction has relaxed (Fig. 4.18). Late decelerations are almost always abnormal, and are indicative of fetal distress.

FETAL BLOOD SAMPLING

Fetal blood sampling (FBS) is a useful tool for the diagnosis of fetal distress. The fetal scalp is visualised with the aid of an amnioscope inserted into the mother's vagina (Fig. 4.19). Once visualised, the fetal scalp is cleaned with a swab, then sprayed with ethyl chloride to induce hyperaemia. A small cut is then made in the fetal scalp, and fetal blood collected in a microtube for immediate analysis.

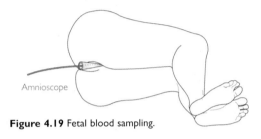

Amnioscope

Figure 4.19 Fetal blood sampling.

A pH value > 7.25 is regarded as normal. A pH value of 7.20–7.25 is regarded as borderline; guidance is to repeat the fetal blood sample within 45 minutes if delivery is not accomplished within that time-frame.

A pH value < 7.20 represents significant fetal hypoxia and the fetus will be distressed. Delivery should take place using the fastest means possible, either by instrumental delivery or by caesarean section.

Indications for fetal blood sampling are as follows:

- Prolonged loss of baseline variability on CTG.

- Persistent late decelerations on CTG.

- Persistent fetal tachycardia.

- Grade 2 or 3 meconium stained liquor, if the CTG is suspicious or the labour is prolonged.

Contra-indications to fetal blood sampling are as follows:

- Known maternal blood-borne infection, such as HIV or hepatitis B.

- Known maternal genital infection such as genital herpes.

MECONIUM

Meconium is fetal faeces. It is rarely produced pre-term, but present in one-third of post-date deliveries. Because meconium can be passed under normal circumstances, its presence is not a reliable indicator of fetal compromise. Similarly, the absence of meconium is not a reliable indicator of fetal well-being; sometimes the fetal head obstructs the flow of meconium out of the vagina thus hiding it from the midwife.

If the meconium is old or dilute it may not be significant; if it is thick or undiluted, then it is often passed in response to hypoxia. A hypoxic fetus will make involuntary gasping movements, and inhale meconium. In these situations, the risk of perinatal death is increased 4-fold and, if the baby survives, it may develop meconium aspiration syndrome. For these reasons, it is important to establish, either by CTG interpretation or with a fetal blood sample, that a fetus that has passed meconium in utero is not hypoxic before allowing labour to continue.

ABNORMAL LABOUR

PRE-TERM LABOUR

Pre-term labour is defined as labour that occurs before 37 weeks of gestation. Pre-term labour results in babies being born who are premature, and of low birth-weight. Neonatal deaths and long-term handicap can result, particularly if labour occurs prior to 32 weeks' gestation. There are over 8000 very low weight babies (under 1500 g) born each year in the UK; these babies are prone to multiple complications.

There are a number of precipitants that can lead to the onset of pre-term labour. These include fetal abnormality, drug abuse, maternal trauma, and infection. If there has been premature rupture of membranes, oral steroids are given to the mother to help mature the fetal lungs by stimulating the production of surfactant in preparation for early birth. There are some circumstances when a myometrial relaxant, such as Atosiban, is given to the mother to try to post-pone labour. There is no clear evidence that these drugs reduce mortality, but they may provide the few key hours of delay required for the fetal lungs to produce enough surfactant to be able to breath once born, or can buy time to get the mother to an obstetric unit for a safe delivery.

INDUCTION AND AUGMENTATION OF LABOUR

Induction of labour is the artificial stimulation of labour when it has not yet started spontaneously. In 2008, approximately one in five UK labours were induced.

INDICATIONS FOR INDUCTION OF LABOUR

Post-dates: NICE guidance states that induction of labour should be offered to all women between the gestation time of 41+0 and 42+0 weeks of gestation in order to avoid the risks of prolonged pregnancy.

Intra-uterine death: if intra-uterine death occurs before term, labour may not start spontaneously. A dead fetus poses a high risk of infection, sepsis, and disseminated intravascular coagulation to the mother if left in situ; it must, therefore, be delivered as soon as conveniently and safely possible. An induced vaginal delivery has the fewest complications and is the preferred method of delivery. If the mother is mentally unable to cope with a vaginal delivery, caesarean section may be offered.

Maternal complications: any maternal complication that requires urgent treatment and delivery of the fetus is a rea-son for induction of labour. Such situations include pre-eclampsia or eclampsia, decompensating cardiac failure, uncontrollable diabetes, or malignancy, to name but a few. Note that maternal request is not an indication for induc-tion of labour prior to 41 weeks' gestation. However, under exceptional circumstances (for example, if the woman's partner is soon to be posted abroad with the armed forces), induction may be considered at or after 40 weeks.

Fetal complications: fetal complications such as severe intra-uterine growth restriction, fetal compromise (such as twin–twin transfusion syndrome), or placental insufficiency are all indicators for induction of labour.

BISHOP SCORE TO ASSESS ONSET OF LABOUR

The Bishop score is a pre-labour scoring system (Table 4.1) that is used to assist in the assessment of labour induction. The Bishop score is made up of five components as follows. The highest possible score is thirteen.

Table 4.1 Bishop score to assess onset of labour

	Bishop score			
	0	1	2	3
Cervical position	Posterior	Intermediate	Anterior	–
Cervical consistency	Firm	Intermediate	Soft	–
Cervical effacement	0–30%	40–50%	60–70%	80%
Cervical dilation	Closed	1–2 cm	2–3 cm	> 3 cm
Fetal station	−3	−2	−1, 0	+1, +2

- *Bishop score < 5* – a score under five is 'unfavourable' indicating that labour is not likely to start spontaneously, and induction is less likely to be successful.
- *Bishop score 8–9* – a score of over seven is 'favourable'. In these women the cervix is said tobe ripe.
- *Bishop score > 9* – a score of over nine suggests that labour is close approaching.

WAYS OF INDUCING LABOUR

'Natural ways' to induce labour

All nulliparous women should be offered a membrane sweep at their 40-week check. This involves the midwife or obstetrician putting a finger into the cervix, and attempting to separate the amniotic membranes from the base of the uterus. It can be quite uncomfortable. All women, regardless of parity, should be offered a membrane sweep at their 41-week check. There is no clear evidence that sexual intercourse helps in inducing the onset of labour, but can be tried, as can nipple stimulation by the woman's partner (or indeed herself), which will cause some oxytocin release.

Amniotomy

If the cervix has dilated enough that the amniotic membranes can be ruptured artificially, this should be done. Amniotomy in itself may induce the onset of labour, as the fetal head presses more directly onto the cervix, which is no longer cushioned by amniotic fluid, forcing it to dilate.

Pharmacological induction of labour

Pharmacological induction of labour cannot take place at home as it carries too many risks; therefore, arrangements need to be made for the woman to be admitted onto the obstetric unit before any chemical inducing agent is given. She is then examined, the fetal heart auscultated, and a Bishop score taken.

Vaginal prostaglandin, such as dinoprostone, is the preferred method used to induce labour chemically. When the decision has been made to induce labour, one dose of prostaglandin (vaginal tablet, gel, or slow-release pessary) is put into the posterior fornix of the vagina. Six hours later, the Bishop score is re-assessed and, if required, a second dose of prostaglandin can be administered (this is not required with the slow-release pessary).

Once labour has started, intravenous oxytocin (Syntocinon) can be given to augment labour. Syntocinon cannot be used if the cervix is not ripe, and cannot be used to start labour.

Contra-indications to pharmacological induction of labour are grand-multiparity, multiple pregnancy, placenta praevia and previous caesarean section.

RISKS OF PHARMACOLOGICAL INDUCTION OF LABOUR

Induced labour is recognised to be more painful than spontaneous labour and there is a much higher need for assisted delivery. In worse case scenarios, pharmacological induction of labour can cause uterine hyperstimulation, uterine rupture, or cord prolapse. Any of these sequelae will cause the fetus to become distressed and, if the situation is uncontrolled, the fetus can die.

Induction of labour may fail; the cervix can refuse to dilate and the uterus may or may not contract. However, the reason that induction was deemed to be necessary remains. As such, the obstetrician may feel compelled to carry out an elective caesarean section, even though neither the fetus nor mother show any signs of distress. The decision to induce labour must, therefore, be taken very seriously indeed.

OBSTRUCTED LABOUR

Obstructed labour means that, in spite of strong contractions of the uterus, the fetus cannot descend through the pelvis because there is an insurmountable barrier preventing its descent. It is crucial to identify the cause of obstruction early in labour, so as to take the appropriate action. Failure to progress is often the earliest sign of obstructed labour. As the time spent labouring becomes prolonged, the mother will tire and the fetus will begin to show signs of distress.

The three 'Ps' as the causes of obstruction of labour

The causes of obstructed labour are often described as being due to three 'Ps':

Powers – obstruction is due to poor or unco-ordinated uterine action.

Passenger – obstruction is due to a large fetal head or abnormal position. Malpresentation is the most common cause for obstructed labour. Fetal hydrocephalus or locked twins are rare causes.

Passage – obstruction due to an abnormally shaped pelvis or an obstruction in the pelvis (such as a pelvic tumour or a large uterine fibroid) will cause arrest in the first stage of labour. This is because the fetal head will be held back at the pelvic inlet, and as such is unable to exert pressure on the cervix to make it dilate. An obstruction in the birth canal, such as cervical or vaginal stenosis, or female genital mutilation causing a tight introitus can also cause arrest of the second stage of labour.

In selected cases, Syntocinon can be useful to strengthen uterine contractions and thereby aid flexion and rotation of the fetal head.

Effect of obstructed labour on fetus

Due to pressure from the cervix as the head passes through the birth canal, the flexible bones of the fetal skull overlap and mould. This facilitates the passage of the fetus through the birth canal, but the moulding can cause formation of a lump on the baby's head known as caput succedaneum. This is often seen during normal labour. Caput succedaneum usually self-resolves over the first few hours and days of the neonatal period; however, with prolonged labour, excessive moulding can lead to tears in the meninges, resulting in intracerebral haemorrhage and possible fetal death.

MALPOSITION

Malpositions are abnormal positions of the vertex of the fetal head relative to the maternal pelvis. It is important to assess the position of the fetal head using vaginal examination to feel for the bony land-marks of the anterior fontanelle and saggital suture (Fig. 4.2). In some, but not all, fetuses, a posterior fontanelle is also present.

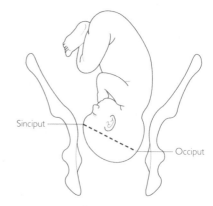

The occiput (Fig. 4.20) is used as a reference point. Occipito-anterior (OA) position is when the occiput is close to the mother's mons pubis. Occipitoposterior (OP) position is when the occiput is close to the mother's anus. When the occiput is close to one or other of the mother's ischial spines, the position is called left or right occipito-transverse (OT).

Figure 4.20 Use of the occiput as a reference point.

In 90% of deliveries, the fetal head is in OA position; in such a position, the fetus naturally flexes its head as it navigates through the pelvis and has a very good chance of being delivered normally. However, some women have a small pelvis, yet carry a big baby. This is known as cephalopelvic disproportion, and is another cause of obstructed labour.

In 10% of deliveries, the fetal head enters the pelvis in OP or OT position; such fetuses are less likely to deliver spontaneously as they are more likely become obstructed as they attempt to descend through the pelvis. This is because in OP or OT position, the longest part of the fetal head is trying to push past the narrowest part of the pelvis. Such deliveries often need instrumental assistance.

COMPLICATIONS OF PROLONGED OBSTRUCTED LABOUR

Fistula formation

When the fetal head is stuck in the pelvis for a very long time, portions of the bladder, cervix, vagina and rectum are trapped between the fetal head and the pelvic bones and subjected to great pressure. The blood supply to those tissues becomes impaired, leading to necrosis. If pressure is maintained over a number of hours or even days, a fistula will form. The fistula may be vesicovaginal (between the bladder and the vagina) or rectovaginal (between the rectum and the vagina).

Puerperal sepsis

Infection is another serious danger for the mother and fetus if labour is prolonged, especially if the amniotic membrane ruptures early. The risk of developing infection is increased by repeated vaginal examinations.

Still-birth

If obstructed labour is allowed to continue indefinitely, the fetus will eventually die. The dead fetus then softens and decomposes, which triggers disseminated intravascular coagulation in the mother. This can cause maternal haemorrhage, shock and death if not treated.

MANAGEMENT OF OBSTRUCTED LABOUR

EPISIOTOMY

An episiotomy is a surgical incision through the perineum made to enlarge the vagina and assist child-birth (Fig. 4.21). The incision can be midline or at an angle from the posterior end of the vulva, and can be performed with or without local anaesthetic. All episiotomies must be sutured together immediately following delivery in order to secure the best outcome for the mother. The routine use of episiotomy during child-birth has lost favour in recent years as there is little evidence to support the previous claims that it is preferable to a natural perineal tear. Indications for episiotomy include: (i) a rigid perineum that is obstructing vaginal delivery; (ii) the clinician senses that a large tear is imminent; (iii) instrumental deliveries; (iv) shoulder dystocia; and (v) breech delivery.

Episiotomy rate

In the UK, episiotomy occurs in approximately 20% of deliveries; in some countries, particularly in South America, and Eastern Europe, episiotomy may be carried out without maternal consent with rates as high as 99%.

Episiotomy can lead to a number of complications including perineal pain, infection and haemorrhage in the post-partum period, and anal sphincter dysfunction with possible faecal incontinence in the long term.

Long-term effects of episiotomy

Chronic dyspareunia is a problem for some women who have undergone episiotomy. This is partly due to tightening of the introitus following perineal repair, and partly due to the erectile tissues of the vulva being replaced by fibrous tissue.

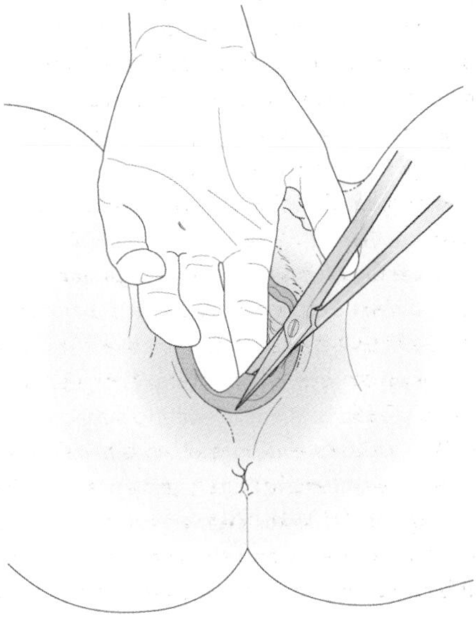

INSTRUMENTAL DELIVERY

Figure 4.21 Mediolateral episiotomy.

There are a number of criteria that must be met prior to attempting an instrumental delivery. These criteria are:

- Labour is obstructed, and delivery unlikely without assistance.
- The fetal head is not palpable above the symphysis pubis.
- The position of the fetal head is known.

- The cervix is fully dilated.
- The amniotic membranes have ruptured.
- The maternal bladder is empty (this can be done by catheterisation).
- Analgesia is satisfactory.
- The clinician has sufficient experience.

If these criteria are not met, caesarean section is indicated.

FORCEPS DELIVERY

There are different types of forceps; some, such as Wrigleys, are used when the head is low lying (*i.e.* on the perineum) and others, such as Neville Barnes, are used when the head is mid-cavity. Kielland's forceps may be used to rotate the fetal head to an OA position. Once the forceps are applied, the obstetrician uses gentle downward traction to deliver the fetus (Fig. 4.22). Incorrect application of the forceps can cause severe trauma to the birth canal and fetal injuries, including facial nerve damage.

VENTOUSE DELIVERY

The ventouse has become increasingly popular as an instrumental method in the UK over recent years, being chosen over the forceps in many cases. A cup is placed on the head of the fetus and suction is applied; then, with the next uterine contraction, downward traction is applied to the cup while the mother pushes (Fig. 4.23). The risk of fetal injury is increased with longer duration of application. Fetal injuries due to use of the ventouse include retinal haemorrhage (if the ventouse cup can been placed incorrectly) and cephalhaematoma.

CAESAREAN SECTION

Caesarean section is the term given to surgical delivery of the fetus via abdominal incision. In the vast majority of cases, the incision is to the lower uterine segment, and so is known as 'lower segment caesarean section' (sometimes seen in the medical notes as LSCS). The alternative to this is the 'classical caesarean section' which involves a vertical uterine incision. This incision is

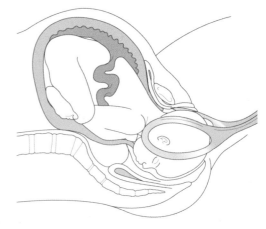

Figure 4.22 Forceps delivery.

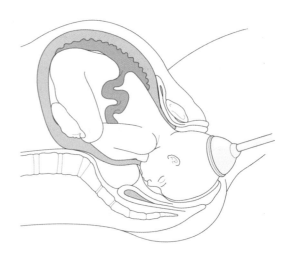

Figure 4.23 Ventouse delivery.

chosen for very pre-term deliveries (when the lower segment of the uterus is not yet fully formed), for those with large lower segment uterine fibroids, or with very anterior placenta praevias.

Elective and emergency caesarean section

A caesarean section can be carried out as an elective or emergency procedure depending on the urgency of the situation. Elective procedures have the best outcome for both mother and baby, and can be done under regional anaesthesia. This allows the mother to be awake throughout the procedure and the baby can be delivered immediately onto her chest. Elective caesarean sections are carried out before the onset of labour. Indications for an elective caesarean section include a previous section, pre-eclampsia, multiple pregnancy, maternal HIV infection or a primary genital herpes infection. Emergency caesarean sections are categorised according to their urgency:

Category 1 – there is an immediate risk to the life of mother or baby. These are so called 'crash sections' and delivery of the fetus is required immediately.

Category 2 – there is evidence of maternal or fetal compromise. Such sections are usually required within an hour, these are known as 'emergency sections'.

Category 3 – delivery is required but there is no immediate risk to mother or baby.

Category 4 – delivery can be planned for the convenience of patient and staff. These are referred to as elective sections, such as for mothers who have undergone previous caesarean sections, twin pregnancies, or placenta praevia.

Risks associated with caesarean section

A caesarean section is a major operation and, as such, carries associated risks. These include the risk of anaesthetic, haemorrhage, deep vein thrombosis and infection. Postoperative adhesions may form which can cause chronic pelvic pain. The wound can be painful for some weeks during the healing process, and women are advised not to drive after their operation for some weeks (a rule of thumb is that she can drive again when she can stamp her foot on the ground without wincing in pain). Postoperative adhesions may form which can cause chronic pelvic pain. A prior caesarean section confers a risk of uterine rupture of 1 in 200 during subsequent labour.

OTHER SERIOUS COMPLICATIONS OF DELIVERY

PLACENTAL ABRUPTION

Placental abruption (also known as abruptio placentae) is the term given to the situation when the placenta separates from the uterus prior to delivery. Placental abruption is suspected when a pregnant woman has sudden, localised, uterine pain with or without bleeding. On examination, the uterus will feel tense and rigid to palpation; there will be maternal tachycardia and postural blood pressure drop if there has been significant blood loss. The fundus may rise if a collection of blood is forming. An ultrasound scan can be used to rule out placenta praevia, but is not diagnostic for abruption.

Risk factors for development of placental abruption

There are several known risk factors that predispose to the occurrence of placental abruption, these are as follows:

- *Maternal trauma*, such as motor vehicle accidents, assaults, falls.

- *Drug use*, particularly tobacco, alcohol, and cocaine.

- *Short umbilical cord.*

- *Prolonged rupture of membranes* (> 24 hours).

- *Maternal age*: pregnant women who are younger than 20 years or older than 35 years are at greater risk.

- *Previous abruption*: women who have had an abruption in previous pregnancies are at greater risk.

Symptoms and signs of placental abruption

Placental abruption typically presents as a painful, hard uterus, in an unwell woman with or without vaginal bleeding. Bleeding always occurs with placental abruption, but it may occur behind the placenta and so is not released from the vagina – the so-called 'concealed abruption'. Bleeding may be from maternal and/or fetal circulations, and so both mother and fetus can become severely compromised. In these cases, urgent attendance to the labour ward is required for resuscitation and emergency delivery.

Management of placental abruption

Immediate management is important; this involves assessing the airway, breathing and circulation of what may be a collapsed mother. The next step is to take basic observations, gain intravenous access, and draw off blood for analysis and cross-match as the mother may need intravenous fluids or a blood transfusion to ensure haemodynamic stability.

Treatment depends on the amount of maternal blood loss and the status of the fetus. Fetal compromise must be assessed by timing the fetal heart rate. If the fetus is less than 36 weeks' gestation and neither mother nor fetus is in any distress, then the mother can be admitted to hospital and observed. If the mother is in shock or the fetus is in distress, then immediate delivery of the fetus is required. Vaginal birth is preferred over caesarean section if there is time. If mother or fetus become compromised, then an emergency caesarean section may be necessary.

SHOULDER DYSTOCIA

Shoulder dystocia occurs after the delivery of the fetal head when the anterior shoulder becomes arrested, lodged behind the symphysis pubis. Normal, gentle, downward traction and episiotomy should be enough to manoeuvre the anterior shoulder out of the birth canal; however, in shoulder dystocia, this is not sufficient and the baby can become well and truly stuck in the birth canal (Fig. 4.24). Note that strong downward traction should never be used as this simply results in an Erb's palsy (a motor paralysis affecting C5–C6) or Klumpke's palsy (a motor paralysis affecting C7–T1) in the neonate. Once the head is delivered, the umbilical cord is tightly compressed in the birth canal. This can prevent the flow of blood to and from the fetus, and yet the fetus is unable to take its first breath as the lungs are also compressed. There is, therefore, only limited time to deliver the fetal body once the head is out before brain injury or death results. Shoulder dystocia is one of the most frightening obstetric emergencies.

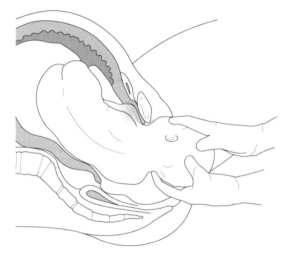

Figure 4.24 Shoulder dystocia.

GOOD PRACTICE POINT 4.3

- Shoulder dystocia is an emergency and requires full obstetric and midwifery team assistance. If you are on a labour ward or delivery suite, pull the emergency red cord to summon help as soon as shoulder dystocia is noticed. If you are at a home birth try the manoeuvres below and get a relative to call an ambulance with full neonatal support as soon as possible.

Risk factors for shoulder dystocia

There are well-recognised risk factors for the development of shoulder dystocia, such as: (i) maternal diabetes; (ii) fetal macrosomia; (iii) maternal obesity; (iv) high parity; and (v) previous dystocia. However, each of these risk factors has only very limited predictive value; over half of all shoulder dystocias occur in normal-sized fetuses and 98% of large fetuses do not have dystocia.

Management of shoulder dystocia

There are a number of obstetric manoeuvres described to manage this emergency, and effective teamwork is essential; the emergency crash team (or whoever is available if the delivery is not in hospital) must be summoned immediately.

- The maternal pelvis should be widened by forced flexing and abducting the hips hard against the abdomen (this usually requires one midwife/doctor pushing upwards on each knee), and telling the mother to push; Fig. 4.25).

- One should attempt to deliver the posterior arm. This allows more room for the anterior shoulder to come under the symphysis.

- Episiotomy and downward traction.

- Suprapubic pressure attempts to push the anterior fetal shoulder under the symphysis pubis (Fig. 4.26).

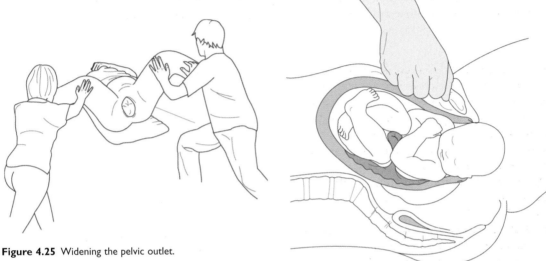

Figure 4.25 Widening the pelvic outlet.

Figure 4.26 Suprapubic pressure over anterior fetal shoulder.

Most cases of shoulder dystocia will be delivered if the above are done properly; if not, deliberate fracture of the fetal anterior clavicle or division of the maternal pelvis symphysis can be carried out as last resort methods.

It is important that all manoeuvres used, and the fetal position, are documented accurately, as the management of shoulder dystocia can be a cause of litigation. There have been recognised cases where brachial plexus injury affects the posterior arm (i.e. not the one that was stuck under the pubic symphysis) because it has got stuck on the sacral promontory. In those cases, no one can be said to be at fault. That is why clear and complete documentation (e.g. which way the baby's head was facing and, therefore, which arm was stuck under the symphysis, etc.) is wise.

CORD PROLAPSE

Cord prolapse is the term given to the situation when the umbilical cord presents first, before the fetus. The prolapsed cord may be visible protruding from the vagina, or may be found on vaginal examination in response to CTG abnormality. This is an obstetric emergency as the prolapsed cord, once exposed to the cold outside environment, can go into spasm (this is an important physiological mechanism for stopping blood flow between baby and placenta post-delivery). This cuts off the oxygen supply to the fetus, which is still in the birth canal. Direct pressure of the fetal body against the umbilical cord is another factor that restricts oxygen supply to the fetus.

Predisposing factors to development of cord prolapse
Predisposing factors include breech presentation, prematurity, long umbilical cord, artificial rupture of membranes and being a second twin.

Management of cord prolapse

Once cord prolapse has been identified, the fetus (if still alive) must be delivered by the quickest means possible. This may be by instrumental delivery if in the second stage of labour, or crash caesarean section if in the first stage of labour. While being transferred to theatre, the mother should be on all fours, in 'knee to chest' position (Fig. 4.27), with a midwife's hand in the vagina pushing the fetal head away from the introitus and thus relieving pressure on the prolapsed cord.

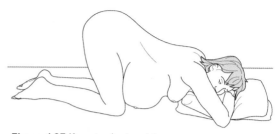

Figure 4.27 Knee-to-chest position.

BREECH PRESENTATION

Breech presentation describes a fetus that is not presenting with the head. There are three main types:

- *Flexed breech* – the hips are flexed with the thighs against the chest; the knees are flexed so that the feet are by the buttocks (Fig. 4.28).

- *Extended or frank breech* – the hips are flexed with the thighs against the chest; the knees are extended so that the feet are by the ears (Fig. 4.29).

- *Footling breech* – a foot, rather than the buttocks, is the presenting part, with one or both feet lying below the buttocks.

Pre-disposing factors to breech presentation

Breech presentation is associated with multiple pregnancy, bicornate uterus, fibroid uterus, placenta praevia, polyhydramnios, fetal neural tube defects, and autosomal trisomies.

Fetuses that present breech can be successfully delivered vaginally by an experienced midwife or obstetrician. However, breech deliveries do carry more risks than cephalic presenting deliveries. Breech deliveries carry higher risk of umbilical cord prolapse, fetal hypoxia, spinal cord transaction, and wide-spread bruising. For these reasons, if the fetus is in a breech position at 38 weeks' gestation, an attempt at external cephalic version is offered. This involves giving a myometrial relaxant, such as ritodrine, and trying to roll the baby round by applying abdominal pressure. If external cephalic version fails, elective caesarean section is often planned. The wishes of the mother must be taken into consideration when making this decision.

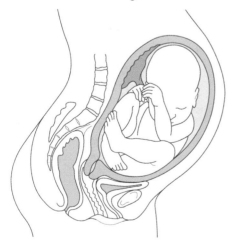

Figure 4.28 Breech presentation (flexed).

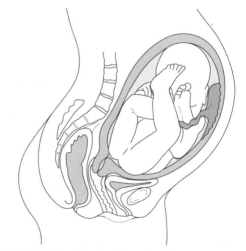

Figure 4.29 Breech presentation (frank).

POST-PARTUM HAEMORRHAGE

It is normal for women to lose some blood during, and immediately following, delivery; this is usually between 200–300 ml. Postpartum haemorrhage (PPH) is the loss of over 500 ml of blood, and is one of the most common causes of maternal death within the developed world. Primary PPH is loss of ≥ 500 ml blood within 24 hours of delivery. Secondary PPH is loss of ≥ 500 ml blood between 24 hours and 6 weeks of delivery.

Causes of post-partum haemorrhage

Causes of postpartum haemorrhage are often referred to under four categories commonly called 'The Four Ts':

T for Trauma – as the fetus passes through the birth canal, the cervix or vagina may sustain lacerations which can bleed quite extensively. The perineum may tear and, in rare cases, the uterus may rupture. If such trauma is not identified early and repaired, significant post-partum bleeding can result.

T for Tone – this refers to the situation when there is insufficient ability of the uterus to contract due to atony. Efficient uterine contraction is not only essential in order to successfully expel the fetus, but is also required post delivery in order to achieve haemostasis. As soon as the fetus and placenta have been delivered, haemostasis relies on the uterine muscle contracting down and compressing the blood vessels within the myometrium. If the uterus fails to contract properly, there will be continuous bleeding.

T for Tissue – this refers to any cellular debris from the placenta, fetus or membranes that remain within the uterine cavity after delivery. Retained products of conception are a common cause of uterine atony, as the uterus is unable to contract and clamp down as it usually does after labour. It is, therefore, important to check that the placenta has been delivered complete as part of routine post-partum care.

T for Thromboformation – this refers to a failure of the clotting cascade, such as may occur with thrombin disorders, haemophilia or von Willebrand's disease. Disseminated intravascular coagulation can also be a cause of post-partum bleed.

Signs and symptoms of post-partum haemorrhage

Post-partum haemorrhage may be noticed by a continuous vaginal bleed but, in many cases, the bleeding is not obvious as a large volume of blood can pool inside the uterine cavity or vagina where it is unnoticed. In such cases, the woman may present with signs of haemorrhagic shock, pallor, nausea, malaise, tachycardia and a postural blood-pressure drop.

Treatment of post-partum haemorrhage

Treatment of post-partum haemorrhage is urgent. If the bleed is occurring at home delivery, an ambulance needs to be called urgently and the woman transported to hospital for emergency management.

A first-line measure is to use bimanual compression to rub the uterus, and cause it to contract (Fig. 4.30). This simple measure is often very effective. While someone is doing this, another member of the team should obtain intravenous access, draw off some blood for cross-matching, and give intravenous colloid fluids and syntometrine.

The cause of PPH must be found and treated, i.e. a cervical laceration, if present, needs to be sutured. Any retained products from the uterus needs to be removed. Should a coagulation disorder be present, fresh frozen plasma (FFP) may be required. In rare cases, hysterectomy is the only way to control a post-partum haemorrhage.

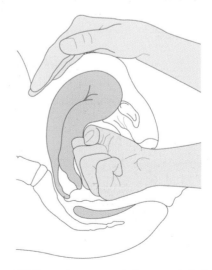

Figure 4.30 Bimanual pressure to 'rub up contraction'

> **GOOD PRACTICE POINT 4.4**
>
> • Causes of post-partum haemorrhage include: (i) trauma (e.g. perineal tear); (ii) tone (e.g. atonic uterus); (iii) tissue (e.g. retained products of conception); and (iv) thrombo-formation (e.g. eclampsia).

CULTURAL AND RELIGIOUS ATTITUDES TO CHILD-BIRTH

Pregnancy and child-birth means so much more to people and families than simply biological reproduction. They are clearly social events, especially so for the nulliparous woman who during pregnancy is in a stage of social transition into the new realm of motherhood. Women react to this change in different ways: some easily assume their new position in society and naturally settle into their new role in the family, whilst others find the change frightening, and feel unprepared, apprehensive or even inadequate to play the role of a mother.

Healthcare workers, particularly the midwife and GP, need to be skilled in recognising vulnerable women and providing extra support where required. However, the huge role that her society, family and religion play during this crucial time of change must be recognised. This influence can be positive and supportive, or dreaded by the pregnant woman, and will profoundly affect the way that she copes with her pregnancy and child-birth. Many cultural practices are disliked by the women involved, but are, nevertheless, strictly adhered to due to expectations from her wider family and community.

There are many cultural taboos that affect post-partum women. The following are a few examples:

- Among traditional Chinese families, new mothers are confined to the house for a period of one month post-delivery.

- African Zulu women are considered dangerous to livestock, plants, and their husbands while they are passing lochia and, as such, are kept in isolation during that time.

- Jehovah's Witnesses will usually refuse all blood and blood products. They should talk to their consultant during their pregnancy about what this implies, and they should be encouraged to provide an advance directive for the hospital notes.

- Orthodox Jewish couples are not allowed any physical contact if the woman is bleeding; once labour starts, whilst the husband may stay with his wife, he will not touch her. This lack of physical contact continues until the woman has had seven clear days without blood loss.

- In some cultures it is traditional to keep the placenta and bury it. Those in Islamic cultures consider the placenta as polluted and will want it to be disposed of quickly.

> **GOOD PRACTICE POINT 4.5**
>
> • Be sensitive to women, their partners, family, and their cultural values.

Module 5:
Postpartum and neonatal care

You will be expected to understand and demonstrate appropriate knowledge, management skills and attitudes in relation to postpartum maternal problems including: the normal and abnormal postpartum period, postpartum haemorrhage, therapeutics, perineal care, psychological disorders, infant feeding and breast problems.

You will be expected to demonstrate an understanding of the investigation and management of immediate neonatal problems including neonatal resuscitation.

This Module focuses on the new born baby and the mother who is recovering from delivery. It provides guidance on successful breast feeding, how to know when lochia is abnormal, and emotional support for the mother. Important neonatal problems are explained.

POST-PARTUM CARE: MANAGEMENT OF NORMAL MINOR PROBLEMS

> **USEFUL WEBSITE**
>
> • NICE Guidance: Postnatal care: routine postnatal care of women and their babies <http://guidance.nice.org.uk/CG37>.

POST-NATAL CHECKS

In the UK, it is customary for post-partum women to attend their GP at 6 weeks after delivery for a routine 'check-up'; many GPs also like to do a check at 2 weeks, which is good practice. Contraception is needed from 3 weeks' post partum unless the woman is very fully breast feeding, not sexually active, or wanting another pregnancy. Post-natal checks usually involve measurement of blood pressure and weight; also, a general assessment of the mother should be made to ascertain how well she is coping with her new baby. The 6-week check is a valuable opportunity for a new mother to ask questions and receive advice, and she should be free to lead the consultation with her agenda, and at her speed. Contraception should be offered, lochia should have stopped, a caesarean section scar should be healing, and the uterus should be well contracted down to pre-pregnancy size. It is prudent to ensure that the mother has been having contact with her health visitor, and that she has an appointment for her baby's first immunisations at 8 weeks.

NORMAL LOCHIA

Lochia is the name for the normal post-partum bloody vaginal discharge. Lochia is typically produced for 4 weeks after delivery and progresses through three stages. The first stage, known as lochia rubra (named after its red colour), is produced for the first 3–5 days. It consists of mainly blood, mucus and placental tissue. The next stage is known as lochia serosa, which lasts for about a week. It is made up of blood, mucus and serous exudate. Lochia alba is the name given to the discharge once it has become a yellowish-white colour, being made up of leukocytes, epithelial cells, cholesterol, fat, and mucus. Lochia alba is produced for about a month.

Lochia is not offensive and passage of lochia should not be painful. If the woman complains that her lochia has a pungent smell or if she is experiencing cramping pains, this probably indicates an infection and, as such, requires treatment with antibiotics. If symptoms persist, she may require an ultrasound scan of the uterus to assess whether retained products of conception are present.

BREAST FEEDING

Caring for and feeding the neonate is an essential part of human reproduction. Both mothers and fathers have a role to play, and this should be encouraged.

Breast milk is recommended as the best source of nutrition for every baby, the only exception being those babies born from HIV-positive mothers. Breast feeding is encouraged to start immediately following delivery of the fetus (there is no need to wait for delivery of the placenta and membranes). The release of oxytocin caused by the baby suckling on the nipples helps the uterus to contract. Women are encouraged to feed their baby 'on demand', which usually works out to be every couple of hours. One breast should be emptied before moving onto the second breast, and each feed should start with the breast that was not emptied at the previous feed. The mother can be re-assured that the baby is getting enough milk if weight gain is adequate and there are wet nappies throughout the day. Breast-fed babies may pass anything between many loose stools a day, to one stool a week, and the mother must be re-assured that this is normal, and encouraged to continue on-demand breast feeding.

Expressing breast milk

Breast milk can be expressed and kept in the fridge for up to 24 hours, or frozen for up to 3 months. This is particularly useful if the mother and baby will be separated for sometime, or if another individual, such as the father or grandmother, would like to feed the baby. A bottle of breast milk is also useful for times when it will be unsuitable for the mother to breast feed (perhaps while out in public or at work), or for premature babies on a neonatal unit (the mother can express milk throughout the day at home, and bring in bottles for the ward). It should be mentioned to mothers that breast milk separates very quickly into fat and whey; therefore, breast milk that has been kept in the fridge needs shaking prior to use.

Medications during breast feeding

There are a number of medications that can be passed to the baby via the mother's breast milk and so it is important that clinicians check all new medications are safe prior to prescribing. Common medications that can be harmful to the breast-fed neonate include ACE inhibitors such as ramipril, calcium channel blockers such as amlodipine, combined hormonal contraceptives such as microgynon 30, Evra and Nuva ring, cytotoxic drugs such as methotrexate, and sedatives such as benzodiazepines or zopiclone. Drugs known to be safe during breast feeding include methyl dopa, paracetamol, progesterone-only contraceptives, penicillin, and senna. Always check in the relevant section of the *BNF*.

Formula feeding

Bottle feeding the infant using formula milk is the alternative to breast feeding, and chosen by many mothers. Although breast feeding is generally preferable, it is important that mothers who choose to formula-feed rather than breast-feed are not made to feel guilty in anyway, and are supported in their decision. There are some benefits to formula feeding, such as allowing the mother to rest or work, allowing the mother to take required medication, and so forth.

It is important that a strict hygiene regimen is adhered to when bottle feeding; the bottles and teats need frequent sterilising, and the milk should be made up from cooled, boiled water. Only one feed should be made at any time, and any left-over milk should be discarded. It cannot be stored, as breast milk can.

Some babies swallow a lot of air while bottle feeding. The mother should be instructed to keep the teat full of milk (rather than half milk, half air) to minimise this problem. The infant should then be 'winded' after a feed, which involves rubbing the baby's back to encourage burping. The baby should never be left with a propped up bottle to suck on as choking can easily occur. Many parents like to warm the milk before giving it to the baby; this is best done by sitting the bottle in warm water. The temperature of the milk should be tested by putting a few drops on the inner surface of the adult's wrist.

Once formula milk has been introduced, the quantity of breast milk produced by the mother will rapidly decrease. If breast feeding has been well established, changing to bottle feeds and weaning the child onto solids can be quite an emotional time for all involved.

SORE NIPPLES

Sore nipples may be caused by *Candida* infection (thrush) which can be treated with a topical antifungal cream, such as clotrimazole, after each feed (the nipples should be wiped prior to feeding to remove the cream). The baby should be checked for oral thrush and treated with oral nystatin drops if present. An alternative is to give the mother miconazole oral gel which can be applied both to the baby's oral mucosa, and to the mother's nipples.

MANAGEMENT OF POST-PARTUM COMPLICATIONS

BABY BLUES

Baby blues is so common that it can be considered normal. Symptoms include being weepy, irritable, and generally feeling low in mood. It usually starts around the third day after delivery and resolves by the tenth day. It does not require any medical treatment, but the beneficial effect of re-assurance and social support should not be underestimated.

ENDOMETRITIS

Endometritis is the term given to inflammation of the endometrium; the most common cause of endometritis is infection. Symptoms include lower abdominal pain, fever and abnormal vaginal bleeding or purulent discharge. Caesarean section, prolonged rupture of membranes, a long labour with multiple vaginal examinations, and retained products of conception are important risk factors. Endometritis can also follow termination of pregnancy, particularly if there was chlamydial or gonococcal infection present. Menstruation after acute endometritis is painful, heavy and offensive. Treatment is with broad-spectrum antibiotics such as co-amoxiclav and metronidazole and, in uncomplicated cases, endometritis will resolve within 2 weeks of treatment. If a sexually transmitted infection is identified, the partner should be notified and treated, and intercourse avoided till at least a week after successful treatment of both partners.

MASTITIS AND BREAST ABSCESSES

Mastitis presents as a painful, red, swollen area of the breast, and can be a complication of a blocked milk duct. Breast feeding should continue, and a good feed on the blocked breast may help relieve engorgement.

A breast abscess may occasionally develop. In such cases, breast feeding should continue from the non-affected breast, and milk should be expressed and discarded from the affected breast until the infection has resolved. An antibiotic such as flucloxacillin or co-amoxiclav may be used safely.

DEEP VEIN THROMBOSIS

Virchow's triad of hypercoagulability, stasis and endothelial injury are all present during pregnancy and the puerperium, therefore the incidence of deep vein thrombosis (DVT) is higher during these periods when incidence is compared to non-pregnant women. The risk of DVT is raised further if the woman is rendered sedentary or immobile following caesarean section.

Deep vein thrombosis usually presents as a painful, swollen, red calf which can spread up the leg to affect the thigh. It is an important diagnosis to make as if untreated the thrombus can embolise through the vena cava, the right side of the heart, all the way to reach the lungs where it will become clogged in one of the smaller vessels. Pulmonary infarction will ensue; if infarction occurs over a sufficiently large area of the lung tissue, sudden unexpected and tragic death of the mother can result from respiratory and cardiac failure.

If DVT is found to be present, treatment is anticoagulation with heparin in the first instance, while a therapeutic level of warfarin is achieved. Warfarin is safe even if breast feeding, and is effective in minimising the risk of pulmonary embolism.

POST-NATAL DEPRESSION

Post-natal depression is said to affect one in ten mothers in the post-partum period, but is grossly under-reported. Having looked forward to having a new baby throughout pregnancy, mothers find it difficult to acknowledge their feelings of despair and persistent low mood, viewing these as contradictory to how they 'should be feeling'. Sufferers have poor sleep, low libido, feelings of poor self-worth and feelings of inability to cope. There may be loss of interest in the baby, irritability, poor concentration, feelings of guilt and inadequacy, and the want to harm the new baby. The depression usually develops at around 4–6 weeks after the delivery, and may persist for many months if not recognised and treated. Very few mothers actually do harm their baby.

Causes of postnatal depression

The cause of postnatal depression is thought to be multifactorial. The sudden decrease in serum progesterone following child-birth may precipitate low mood and irritability in some (in just the same way as it causes premenstrual tension). The new stressful social situation, responsibility, and demands of motherhood may precipitate a depression in women who find this to be a particularly vulnerable time of life. There may be social isolation, financial strain, poor sleep and fatigue which can all accumulate.

Treatment of postnatal depression

The mainstay of treatment involves early recognition, and support from the mother's family and friends, the health visitor, local mother and baby groups, and the GP. This is often all that is required to bring the lady smoothly through this difficult time. In some cases, such as mothers with a previous history of depression or mental illness, an antidepressant may be indicated.

Edinburgh Postnatal Depression Score

The Edinburgh Post-Natal Depression Score (Appendix 5.1) is often used either by the health visitor, or by the GP at the 6-week check, as a quick screening method to pick up mothers suffering from post-natal depression. This scale has possibly lost its usefulness in recent years as mothers are reported to answer questions in order to avoid the diagnosis of depression, or perhaps to try to say 'the right thing' and please the listener. The Edinburgh Postnatal Depression Score is consequently being used less than previously, and there is a recognised need to develop a more subtle scale.

PUERPERAL PSYCHOSIS

Puerperal psychosis is rare, occurring in only 1 in 500 mothers. It is more common if the mother is primiparous, has a psychiatric history, or a family history of mental health illness. Onset is typically within 2 weeks of delivery, presenting with delusions and auditory hallucinations typical of schizophrenic psychosis. The baby is at risk of neglect and harm while the mother is unwell, and may need to be taken into care while the mother is treated. There is some evidence that electroconvulsive therapy is effective in these cases. Relapse, however, is common.

NEONATAL CARE

INITIAL NEWBORN CHECK

Neonates should be examined briefly, immediately after delivery, in order to pick-up any major abnormalities at an early stage. This involves counting the Apgar score, measuring the birth weight, and conducting a brief examination of the face, eyes, mouth, chest, abdomen, spine, limbs and genitalia. Some children may be born with indiscriminate genitalia; in such cases, it is important not to guess at the likely gender of the child, but advise that gender is uncertain and that further tests will be needed.

Apgar score

The Apgar score gives a reproducible, quantitative assessment of neonatal condition that is useful for assessing a baby's progress or deterioration immediately after delivery (Table 5.1). It is important to document the Apgar score in the medical notes for medicolegal reasons. The Apgar score is most useful following complicated or assisted births, or when problems with the baby are anticipated. The score should be checked as soon as the baby is delivered, and at 2 and 5 minutes post delivery.

The maximum Apgar score is ten which describes a very healthy baby. The lowest score is zero, which describes a still-born baby. Apgar score at 5 minutes can be used only with great caution when estimating prognosis.

Table 5.1 Apgar score

	Apgar score		
	0	1	2
Colour of baby	Blue, pale	Body pink, extremities blue	Completely pink
Respiratory effort	Absent	Weak cry, hypoventilation	Good, strong cry and adequate breaths
Muscle tone	Limp	Some flexion of extremities	Active motion with extremities well flexed
Response to plantar stimulation	No response	Grimace	Cry
Heart rate	Absent	Slow (< 100 bpm)	Fast (> 100 bpm)

NEONATAL CHECK

All neonates should receive a full check before their discharge from hospital, or within 72 hours for home births or rapid discharges from birthing units. GPs are responsible for the neonatal checks of babies delivered in the community. A complete neonatal check should involve examining the following:

- Head shape and circumference, presence of anterior fontanelle and whether normal, sunken or bulging.
- Facial appearance and any dysmorphic features.

- Eye shape and appearance. Presence of the red retinal reflex, any signs of ophthalmic infection.

- Ear shape and size, patency of external auditory meatus.

- Deficiency of the soft or hard palate. Sucking reflex.

- Arms, legs, feet and hand shape and symmetric movement. Any evidence of traction birth injury (such as Erb's palsy). Ten fingers and ten toes, palmar creases.

- Presence of brachial, radial and femoral pulses.

- Heart sounds, any added sounds or murmurs.

- Bilateral air entry sounds, and any signs of respiratory distress.

- Abdominal shape, umbilical stump, external genitalia (presence of both testicles in the scrotum of male babies). Presence of an anus and whether meconium has been passed.

- Deficiency of the spine or unusual tufts of hair (i.e. spina bifida).

- Congenital dislocation of the hip.

- Tone, posture, and neonatal reflexes.

NEWBORN HEARING TEST

The newborn hearing test is offered to all babies in the UK within their first month of life. The newborn hearing test is a screening test based on the detection of oto-acoustic emissions (OAE) given off by the tympanic membrane. A probe placed in the baby's ear detects these emissions, which are given off by babies who can hear. If there is an inadequate response, the neonate will be referred for an auditory brainstem response test, which provides more accurate information.

The auditory brainstem response test involves playing sounds to the baby via earphones while he or she is asleep. A computer then records how the baby responds to those sounds.

NEWBORN HEEL-PRICK TEST

The midwife or health visitor takes a heel-prick blood test between 6–14 days of life to test for inborn errors of metabolism. This test looks for phenylketonuria, sickle cell anaemia, congenital hypothyroidism, cystic fibrosis, and medium chain acyl-CoA dehydrogenase deficiency.

GOOD PRACTICE POINT 5.1

- At the 6-week check, remember to ensure that the neonatal hearing test, and heel prick test have been done, and that the results have been received and acted on accordingly.

NEONATAL 6-WEEK CHECK

At 6 weeks, the results of the newborn hearing tests and heel prick tests should be back, and the results given to the mother if she has not yet received them.

Either the community baby clinic or the GP should carry out a check of the neonate at around 6–8 weeks of age. This check is very much like the newborn check. Weight, length, head circumference should be measured and recorded in the baby's red book, and current measurements should be compared with birth measurements to assess if growth is adequate. The red reflex is looked for, and an assessment made of whether the baby can fix its gaze on an object and follow it. Tone, ability to hold the head briefly, heart sounds, femoral pulses, breathing, spine, reflexes, genitalia are all checked once again.

NEONATAL RESUSCITATION

Although officially in the realm of neonatology, any obstetrician, gynaecologist, GP, paramedic or accident and emergency clinician may find themselves with a mother who delivers a baby unexpectedly in their presence. The baby may be in poor condition, or even dead. If the baby shows signs of life and is known to be over 24 weeks' gestation, immediate resuscitation must take place. If the baby is under this age, resuscitation may not be appropriate, even if signs of life are demonstrated.

NEWBORN LIFE SUPPORT

Newborn life support comprises the following elements.
 • The umbilical cord should be clamped and cut if this can be done safely, and then the neonate rubbed with a towel as soon as possible after birth. This is stimulating, and will encourage breathing. An assessment must then be made as to whether immediate intervention is required. This is done by quickly taking an Apgar score. If the Apgar score is low, the baby should then be wrapped up to conserve heat, and taken with the rescuer who must call for help as first priority. Once help has been summoned, the baby should be brought into a warm room (if outside), and ideally placed under a radiant heater or resuscitaire. If this is not available, cooking foil and a warm towel can be used to wrap the baby as an interim measure while waiting for an ambulance.

 • The airway must be kept open. This is done by placing the baby on its back with the head neither flexed nor extended. Most newborn babies have a relatively large and heavy occiput which tends to flex the neck and occlude the airway. This can be avoided applying chin lift or jaw thrust.

 • If the baby is not breathing properly by 90 seconds, five inflation breaths should be given. If the heart rate was below 100 bpm initially, this rate will rapidly increase as oxygenated blood reaches the heart. If the heart rate does not increase following inflation breaths, then it is very likely that the lungs are not being adequately aerated. In the minority of cases, the baby will need more than just lung aeration.

 • If the heart rate remains slow (less than 60 bpm) or absent following five inflation breaths, despite good passive chest movement in response to the inflation efforts, chest compression should begin. In babies, the most effective way of giving chest compression is to grip the chest in both hands so that two thumbs press on the lower third of the sternum, with the fingers over the spine at the back (Fig. 5.1). The ratio of compressions to inflations in newborn resuscitation is 3:1.

 • The drugs adrenaline, sodium bicarbonate, or 10% dextrose can be considered once a resuscitation team has arrived. These may be administered through an umbilical catheter.

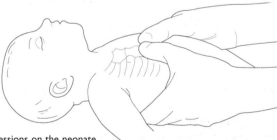

Figure 5.1 Chest compressions on the neonate.

APPENDIX 5.1:

EDINBURGH POST-NATAL DEPRESSION SCORE

As you have recently had a baby, we would like to know how you are feeling.

Please tick the answer which comes closest to how you have felt in the past 7 days, not just how you feel today.

I have been able to laugh and see the funny side of things

☆   *As much as I always could*

☆   *Not quite so much now*

☆   *Definitely not so much now*

☆   *Not at all*

I have looked forward with enjoyment to things

☆   *As much as I ever did*

☆   *Rather less than I used to*

☆   *Definitely less than I used to*

☆   *Hardly at all*

I have blamed myself unnecessarily when things went wrong.

☆   *Yes, most of the time*

☆   *Yes, some of the time*

☆   *Not very often*

☆   *No, never*

I have been anxious or worried for no good reason

☆   *No, not at all*

☆   *Hardly ever*

☆   *Yes, sometimes*

☆   *Yes, very often*

I have felt scared or panicky for not very good reason

☆   *Yes, quite a lot*

☆   *Yes, sometimes*

☆   *No, not much*

☆   *No, not at all*

Things have been getting on top of me

☆   *Yes, most of the time I haven't been able to cope at all*

☆   *Yes, sometimes I haven't been coping as well as usual*

☆   *No, most of the time I have coped quite well*

☆   *No, I have been coping as well as ever*

I have been so unhappy that I have had difficulty sleeping

☆   *Yes, most of the time*

☆   *Yes, sometimes*

☆   *Not very often*

☆   *No, not at all*

I have felt sad or miserable

☆   *Yes, most of the time*

☆   *Yes, quite often*

☆   *Not very often*

☆   *No, not at all*

I have been so unhappy that I have been crying

☆   *Yes, most of the time*

☆   *Yes, quite often*

☆   *Only occasionally*

☆   *No, never*

The thought of harming myself has occurred to me

☆   *Yes, quite often*

☆   *Sometimes*

☆   *Hardly ever*

☆   *Never*

Module 6:
Gynaecological problems

You will be expected to demonstrate appropriate knowledge, management skills and attitudes in relation to benign gynaecological problems including: urogynaecology, paediatric and adolescent gynaecology, endocrine problems, pelvic pain and abnormal vaginal bleeding. This will include knowledge of early pregnancy loss, including clinical features, investigation and management of disorders leading to early pregnancy loss: miscarriage (including recurrent), ectopic pregnancy and molar pregnancy.

You will be expected to demonstrate an ability to assess and manage common sexually transmitted infections including HIV/AIDS and be familiar with their modes of transmission and clinical features. You will be expected to understand the principles of contact tracing.

You will also be expected to know the basis of national screening programmes and their local implementation through local care pathways. You will be expected to demonstrate appropriate knowledge of clinical features, investigation and management of premalignant and malignant conditions of the female genital tract. You will be expected to have an understanding of the indications and limitations of screening for premalignant and malignant disease. An understanding of the options available for palliative and terminal care including relief of symptoms and community support will be expected.

This Module attempts to cover a vast area.

- First ambiguous genitalia are covered and the different reasons for this.
- Then, paediatric and adolescent gynaecology is addressed, which explains normal growth and pubertal development, and problems that can occur at this time.
- Sexual maturity brings with it the risk of contraction of sexually transmitted infections (STIs) which are described, along with a description of their treatment and prevention.
- The cervical screening programme, and its crucial importance is covered along with an explanation of cervical cancers. In fact, this module covers the diagnosis and management of all cancers affecting the female reproductive system.
- Menopause and hormone replacement therapy, miscarriage and ectopic pregnancy, heavy menstrual bleeding, and pelvic pain are all described.

PAEDIATRIC GYNAECOLOGY: AMBIGUOUS GENITALIA

There are a number of known causes of ambiguous genitalia. The main ones are discussed below.

MASCULINISATION

INGESTION OF ANDROGENIC STEROIDS

Ingestion by the mother of substances with male hormone activity during pregnancy, such as androgenic steroids taken for 'body building' can cause masculinisation of female genitalia.

ADRENAL TUMOUR

Tumours in the fetus or the mother that produce androgenic hormones will cause masculinisation of female genitalia. This occurs with adrenal tumours.

CONGENITAL ADRENAL HYPERPLASIA

Congenital adrenal hyperplasia is the most common cause of ambiguous genitalia in newborns. Some 95% of cases of congenital adrenal hyperplasia are due to 21-hydroxylase deficiency, which is required for cortisol production. There is low or absent cortisol production (depending on the severity of the enzyme defect) and so the anterior pituitary gland overproduces adrenocorticotropic hormone (ACTH) to try and stimulate cortisol production. The effect of this is simply to cause the adrenals to hyperplase (grow in size), and produce more and more of the cortisol precursor, 17-hydroxypregnenolone. This abundance of precursor is then turned into androgens (instead of cortisol), which masculinise the female genitalia.

Babies with congenital adrenal hyperplasia have a number of other problems, which is why early recognition of ambiguous genitalia using the heel-prick test soon after birth is so important. The lack of cortisol will cause an Addisonian salt-wasting crisis, demonstrated with vomiting, severe dehydration, shock, collapse and death within the first month of life if not recognised and treated.

USEFUL WEBSITES

- Patient Support Group: Living with CAH <www.livingwithcah.com>.

- Society for Endocrinology, represents scientists and clinicians who work with hormones <www.endocrinology.org>.

FEMINISATION

LEYDIG CELL APLASIA

Leydig cell aplasia is a condition in which there is impaired testosterone production. This will result in abnormal genitalia development in XY fetuses, which may look female.

ANDROGEN INSENSITIVITY SYNDROME

See under Genetic abnormalities

5-ALPHA-REDUCTASE DEFICIENCY

5-Alpha-reductase deficiency results in low levels of the active testosterone, dihydrotestosterone. As a result, there is under-virilisation of male genitalia, so much so that the child may be brought up as a female and only present in adolescence when primary amenorrhoea is noticed. At this time, testicular descent and growth may be discovered.

PAEDIATRIC GYNAECOLOGY: FOREIGN OBJECT IN THE VAGINA

It is not that uncommon for young girls to poke something in their vagina, just as they may poke something in their ear canal or nostril. It is usually an innocent gesture of exploring their own body; however, if the foreign body, such as a marble, remains in the vagina, it can cause overgrowth of bacteria, and present to the GP with an offensive vaginal discharge. Such an object may be seen on pelvic X-ray, and may require removal by an experienced gynaecologist under anaesthesia.

ADOLESCENT GYNAECOLOGY

PUBERTY

Puberty refers to the process of physiological, physical and hormonal changes by which a child's body becomes an adult body that should be capable of reproduction. It is a major social event, the climax of which is menarche in the female. This is seen by many cultures as the outward demonstration that a female has reached womanhood, and is ready for adult life, marriage, and motherhood.

Somewhere in the limbic system of the brain, there is thought to be a trigger that decides that the time for puberty has come. This is based on having an adequate nutritional status, hereditary factors, and some environmental influence. The hypothalamus responds by starting to secrete pulses of gonadotrophin releasing hormone (GnRH), which later becomes continuous. The anterior pituitary gland responds to the GnRH by secreting pulses of luteinizing hormone (LH) that becomes cyclical once the menstrual cycle is established.

The primordial follicles within the ovaries respond to the LH pulses by growing and producing oestrogen. The oestrogen has a positive feedback function that further stimulates follicle growth. Oestrogen acts on many different organs of the body and is responsible for most of the physical changes that occur during puberty such as breast development, the growth

Table 6.1 Tanner staging for the physical signs of puberty				
Tanner stage	Breasts	Pubic hair	Growth	Other
Stage 1	Elevation of papilla	No hair	Steady growth, 5–6 cm per year	Ovaries enlarge
Stage 2	Breast bud appears under enlarged areolae	Sparse straight hair along labia	Accelerated growth, 7–8 cm per year	Uterus enlarges, clitoral enlargement, labia become darker
Stage 3	Breast tissue grows beyond areolae	Coarser, curlier and darker hair spreads across mons pubis	Peak velocity growth 8 cm per year	Acne likely, axillary hair grows
Stage 4	Areolae projects above breast tissue forming a mound	Adult pattern hair but no spread to medial thighs	Decelerated growth 5–7 cm per year	Menarche with irregular menstrual periods
Stage 5	Adult breast contour with projection of papilla only	Adult pattern hair with spread to medial thighs	Cessation of growth	Regular menstrual periods

spurt (oestrogen acts synergistically with growth hormone), and female deposition of fat. There is an accompanying rise in the levels of adrenal androgens, which are responsible for the growth of pubic and axillary hair, enlargement of the clitoris, and for development of libido, acne, and the more pungent body odour of an adult.

Physical signs of puberty in the female

The adolescent growth spurt is one of the first signs that puberty is beginning. At an average age of 11–12 years, girls undergo acceleration in growth under the influence of oestrogen and growth hormone. The pelvis widens and adipose tissue is laid down on the buttocks. The uterus grows, and the endometrium becomes more vascular. The breasts grow and develop. Course hair starts to grow in the pubic and axillary areas. The girl then starts to menstruate as discussed below.

The physical signs of puberty occur in a specific sequential order and this has been staged by Tanner (Table 6.1).

MENARCHE

Menarche is the term given for the first menstrual period in a female's life. From both social and medical perspectives, it is often considered to be the central event of female puberty as it signifies the possibility of fertility. However, menarche does not necessarily signal that ovulation has occurred: 80% of girls are anovulatory throughout the first year after menarche. It is the acquisition of regular menstrual cycles that shows that puberty is complete and that fertility has been achieved.

The average age of menarche has been steadily falling in the Western world over the past century, which is thought to be a result of better childhood nutrition. The average age of menarche in the UK is currently 12 years of age, but anything between 9–15 years is considered normal. Obese children often enter puberty earlier than children of normal weight due to increased peripheral oestrogen storage in their adipose tissue.

PUBERTAL DELAY

Investigations for pubertal delay should be considered if there is no development of secondary sexual characteristics by the age of 14 years, or no menarche by the age of 16 years. By far the most common reason for this is simple constitutional delay. In such cases, all stages of development are delayed, and height is appropriate for bone age, which can be assessed by looking at the growth plate on a hand/wrist X-ray. There is often a history of pubertal delay in the mother or elder sisters. If the girl is becoming distressed by being behind her peers, experiencing under-achievement or bullying at school due to pubertal delay, she can be urged into puberty by administration of 2 μg ethinyloestradiol daily. This will encourage growth, and 3–6 months of treatment usually results in the onset of self-perpetuating puberty and no further treatment is required. Higher doses of 10–20 μg daily will cause secondary sexual characteristics to appear, but are seldom required unless there is gonadal failure.

Conditions that cause a low body weight are associated with delayed puberty. Such conditions include anorexia nervosa, malnutrition, and chronic medical diseases such as cystic fibrosis or congenital heart disease. Mental health problems such as severe stress or abuse can cause pubertal delay. Chemotherapy and radiotherapy can both cause iatrogenic primary gonadal failure and failure of puberty. Very rarely, pubertal delay may be caused by a brain tumour, such as craniopharyngioma, or by a congenital gonadotrophin deficiency.

Causes of primary and secondary amenorrhoea are discussed in detail later in this Module.

PRECOCIOUS PUBERTY

Some children with brain tumours or other lesions of the hypothalamus may undergo precocious puberty as a result of early and increased secretion of GnRH. They will become sexually mature at an unusually young age if left untreated.

HYMEN RUPTURE

The hymen is a membrane that covers the vaginal introitus. It is of unknown function, but has great social significance in some cultures as it perforates at the first sexual encounter, resulting in a visible bleed. It is, therefore, used by some as a marker for virginity. There are, however, problems with this; the hymen can rupture due to other reasons apart from having sex, such as during horse riding, tampon use or from innocent trauma to the perineum, such as girls who slip while straddling a fence. In some Arabic countries, private operations are done on girls to restore a perforated hymen prior to marriage, to prevent her embarrassment.

FIRST SEXUAL ENCOUNTER

The first sexual encounter is of great significance to most women. There is a great variation in age at which this may occur. Many cultures and religions promote delay of sexual intercourse until after marriage, and frown on sexual promiscuity. However, it is increasingly being accepted in modern societies that there are some benefits to sexual encounters prior to, or even in preference to, marriage, and that more than one sexual partner is permissible. It is important that an individual decision is made on these matters, including one's own sexual preferences and behaviours, and on what each woman feels is acceptable behaviour in their partner. Most people prefer exclusive intimate relationships and feel hurt when a partner has sex with another, but many share sexual partners in an open fashion and without moral difficulty.

In Western culture there is often lack of discussion between parents and their children on sex, with sexual education being left to schools and sexual health clinics. It is, therefore, difficult for young people to make up their own minds on these matters and girls can be strongly influenced by their peer groups and the media. Young women often have grossly inadequate information on how to manage their new sexuality and expose themselves to unnecessary infections, pregnancies and abuse.

PRIMARY AMENORRHOEA AND ITS CAUSES

Primary amenorrhoea is defined as the absence of menarche by the age of 16 years, and the term is used to describe the situation when adult women have never experienced a menstrual period.

CONSTITUTIONAL DELAY

Constitutional delay is by far the most common cause of primary amenorrhoea. This is more common in Asian women when compared with Caucasian women, and is commonly seen if the child is poorly nourished. The GP should make an initial assessment as to whether there is development of any secondary sexual characteristics such as breasts, axillary or public hair. If puberty is in progress, the patient can be re-assured and allowed to 'watch and wait' for another year. If there is concern that sexual characteristics are not developing and the child is small, a referral to paediatrics may be appropriate. The paediatrician will X-ray the hand to see if there is any delay in bone age; if there is bone delay, this suggests that the delay is simply constitutional. In such cases, there is no need for worry, and the parents and child can be re-assured that puberty will most likely take off in its own time. However, often the child is embarrassed that she is behind her classmates, and would like something to speed things up. Starting on the combined oral contraceptive pill (if there are no contra-indications) often works with good effect, as does administration of 2 µg of ethinyloestradiol daily.

IMPERFORATE HYMEN

Another reason for primary amenorrhoea is that the hymen, a thin membrane that covers the vaginal orifice, is imperforate (i.e. there is no hole in it). Normally, the hymen has a small open area in the middle which allows the passage of menstrual blood. The first time a female has sexual intercourse this hymen is perforated, causing a slight bleed. During the first vaginal delivery, the hymen is perforated further, and only remnants of the hymen can be seen at the vaginal orifice after that time.

An imperforate hymen should be looked for in women who have developed secondary sexual characteristics appropriately, but present with primary amenorrhoea. They may even describe monthly pelvic and vaginal cramps which can be quite severe. This is because the menstrual blood collects in the vagina and uterus, causing pressure and stretching. This menstrual blood is then slowly broken down to be re-absorbed into the body. There may be retrograde menstrual flow of blood out of the ends of the fallopian tubes into the pelvis if bleeding is heavy.

Imperforate hymen is usually quite obvious on examination of the female external genitalia. If an imperforate hymen is found, the young woman will need to be referred to a gynaecologist for hymenal incision. This immediately solves the problem, and there are no long-term complications. The surgeon will try to leave some of the hymen untouched so that the first sexual experience will still be evidenced by a small bleed, which is of great importance to some couples, particularly where virginity is highly valued and perforation of the hymen taken as a representation of that.

Eating disorders

Young women of very low body weight, whether this be due to an eating disorder such as anorexia nervosa, excessive exercise and figure control such as is seen in ballerinas, or whether due to malnutrition, all often experience amenorrhoea. This may be primary or secondary. It is particularly common in young women with a body mass index of less than 18 kg/m^2.

USEFUL WEBSITES

- B-EAT: Beat Eating Disorders <www.b-eat.co.uk>.

- Help an information for eating disorders <www.disordered-eating.co.uk>.

- National Centre for Eating Disorders <www.eating-disorders.org.uk>.

- Royal College of Psychiatrists: information for the public
  <www.rcpsych.ac.uk/mentalhealthinformation/mentalhealthproblems/eatingdisorders.aspx>.

If the woman does have such a low body mass, but other secondary sexual characteristics are present, no gynaecological investigations are required. Hwever, a discussion about weight gain should be held. If the low weight is due to an eating disorder, this will need specialist treatment in its own right. Once treated and a normal body weight gained, a re-assuring sign that recovery has occurred is that menstruation will begin. In professional dancers and athletes, young women with amenorrhoea will often know of fellow students or colleagues who have experienced the same symptoms, and may be quite at ease with it and reluctant to gain weight. This decision of balancing the importance of her career with her health is ideally made with the support of her family and friends.

GENETIC ABNORMALITIES CAUSING PRIMARY AMENORRHOEA

There are a number of genetically inherited conditions that may go unknown until young adulthood when a young woman presents with failure to develop secondary sexual characteristics, or primary amenorrhoea. Such conditions include the following.

TURNER'S SYNDROME

Turner's syndrome is a condition that results from non-dysjunction of the sex chromosomes during anaphase of meiotic cell division resulting in the genotype XO. These individuals only have one sex chromosome (normally people have two), otherwise known as monosomy. This results in a number of subtle abnormalities such as a wide neck, shorter than average stature, and widely spaced nipples, but these abnormalities may have been unnoticed. However, women with Turner's syndrome have shrunken, non-functioning ovaries known as streak ovaries. These ovaries do not produce oestrogen as they should under the influence of FSH, and so puberty is not reached and there will be no menarche. Such young women respond well to the combined oral contraceptive pill (if there are no contra-indications).

An alternative is daily administration of 2 μg ethinyloestradiol but generally a cyclical regimen such as the combined oral contraceptive is preferred in order to avoid endometrial hyperplasia.

KALLMANN'S SYNDROME

Kallmann's syndrome is an X-linked or autosomal recessive disorder with greater penetrance in the male. It expresses itself as hypothalamic hypogonadism. There is lack of GnRH from the hypothalamus; there is, therefore, no stimulus to the anterior pituitary gland to release FSH and LH, and no stimulus to the ovary. Put simply, the ovaries do not produce oestrogen, so there is no puberty and no menarche. These women will need to be managed by a specialist centre as care is quite complex. Since the underlying defect is at the hypothalamic level, optimal treatment is with pulsatile GnRH, which mimics the natural situation. This can be administered by a pump attached to the body throughout the day and night. About 50% of treated patients may achieve pregnancies.

ANDROGEN INSENSITIVITY SYNDROME

Androgen insensitivity syndrome used to be known as testicular feminisation. This is a particularly difficult condition to explain to any patient or parent. The defect is due to inheritance, or a spontaneous mutation in the gene for the androgen receptor which stops it working. The fetus is of XY genotype (*i.e.* male genes) but, as the androgen receptor does not work, the young male fetus cannot respond to testosterone, so develops as a female fetus and, when born, is recognised to be a girl. The child will be brought up as a female and only when puberty is reached (breasts will grow as normal but pubic hair is sparse) will it be recognised that something is wrong as there will be no menstruation. Investigations will show that there are no ovaries and no uterus. The vagina stops blindly half way up. All these individuals are infertile as there is neither production of ovum nor sperm. Treatment should be in a genetic centre as there are a number of associated problems in addition to infertility that can arise.

GOOD PRACTICE POINT 6.1

- Even in the case of supposed primary amenorrhoea, consider whether a pregnancy test is required.

SECONDARY AMENORRHOEA AND ITS CAUSES

Secondary amenorrhoea is defined as the cessation of menstruation for 6 months or more.

Pregnancy as a cause of secondary amenorrhoea

Secondary amenorrhoea is a normal occurrence during pregnancy and continues during breast-feeding. This must be remembered as, whenever a woman of child-bearing age presents with secondary amenorrhoea, a pregnancy test must be done first and foremost, as this is by far the most common cause of cessation of menstrual periods.

GOOD PRACTICE POINT 6.2

- If a young girl attends with her mother or friend, still be alert to the need for a pregnancy test. She may need to be seen on her own.

Contraception as a cause of secondary amenorrhoea

Secondary amenorrhoea may occur with many of the contraceptive methods available. These include the contraceptive implant, progestogen-only injectables, the intra-uterine system and the progesterone-only pill. If a woman with secondary amenorrhoea is using one of these contraceptive methods, she can be re-assured that the absence of periods can occur as a result of the contraception itself. She can be informed that the absence of periods is not dangerous to her in any way, and is not a sign that anything is wrong; in fact, it is a good sign that the contraceptive method is working well for her. She can be encouraged to continue on that contraceptive method. There are some women who are not comfortable without the reassurance of a monthly period, and these women may need to change their contraceptive method in order to feel at ease.

Menopause as a cause of secondary amenorrhoea

Secondary amenorrhoea is a normal, natural occurrence that happens when a woman's time of fertility is passed; this is known as reaching the menopause. The menopause will be discussed in detail in Module 8.

Other causes of secondary amenorrhoea

Certain drugs can cause secondary amenorrhoea, such as antipsychotics and immunosuppressants.

Almost any chronic illness can cause menstrual periods to stop. Identification of these is the skill of all good GPs. Often, none of the female reproductive organs are at fault but rather another part of the body will require investigation. Particular diseases that precipitate cessation of menstruation which should be considered include thyroid disease, endocrine tumours, stress, anxiety or depression.

Weight loss for whatever reason can cause secondary amenorrhoea.

ADULT GYNAECOLOGY

PELVIC PAIN DUE TO THE MENSTRUAL CYCLE

For details of the menstrual cycle, please see Module 1.

MITTELSCHMERZ PAIN

Mittelschmerz pain is felt mid-menstrual cycle and is due to ovulation. The pain is often described as coming on quite suddenly and then gradually subsiding over the next few hours, although it can linger for a couple of days. In some women, the pain is localised enough indicate which of the two ovaries produced an ovum in any given month. Because the side on which ovulation is achieved alternates from left to right randomly, the pain may switch sides or stay on the same side from one menstrual cycle to another.

If the history is clear, the woman can be re-assured that Mittelschmerz pain is not harmful and does not signify the presence of any sort of disease. It the menstrual cycles are regular and the pain can be predicted, simple analgesia may be suggested. If the Mittelschmerz pain is a persistent troublesome problem each month, and the woman would like to stop it, a contraceptive method that suppresses ovulation can be offered such as the combined contraceptive pill, Cerazette or the contraceptive implant.

DYSMENORRHOEA

Dysmenorrhoea is the term given for excessively painful periods. Most women find periods painful and many will take simple analgesia (such as ibuprofen or paracetamol), or use simple methods such as holding a hot water bottle on the pelvis. By using such methods, the majority of women adequately manage their pain and are able to function normally while menstruating. For some women, however, such methods are not successful and they may suffer pelvic cramps, nausea, lower back pain and headaches causing time off work or school.

Primary dysmenorrhoea

Primary dysmenorrhoea is idiopathic and typically accompanies periods soon after menarche. There are higher levels of prostaglandins in the menstrual fluid of women suffering from dysmenorrhoea, and it is thought that prostaglandins causing increased uterine contractility are the cause of menstrual pain. As such, NSAIDs (such as mefenamic acid or ibuprofen) are often very effective and are used as first-line treatment. If these fail, suppression of ovulation by use of the combined oral contraceptive pill is also very effective as long as it is not contra-indicated. Injectable progestogens such as Depo-provera are also effective as they may result in amenorrhoea or very light bleeds. The levonorgestrel intra-uterine system is another effective management option.

GOOD PRACTICE POINT 6.3

- Do not underestimate how painful dysmenorrhoea can be. Show empathy and understanding, and refer to a gynaecologist when necessary. Consider referral to cognitive behavioural therapy for selected cases as there is evidence that pain can be managed well using these techniques.

Secondary dysmenorrhoea

Secondary dysmenorrhoea is the development of painful periods which were not previously painful, and is usually due to an underlying cause. A common cause is the intra-uterine device; prior to insertion of these devices, all women should be advised that they may develop more painful periods. Other causes of secondary dysmenorrhoea include pelvic inflammatory disease, caesarean section or other pelvic surgery that can precipitate the formation of pelvic adhesions. These can be very difficult to manage.

ADENOMYOSIS

Adenomyosis is a condition characterised by the presence of ectopic endometrial tissue within the myometrium. The condition is typically found in women between the ages of 35–50 years. Patients with adenomyosis can suffer from both dysmenorrhoea and menorrhagia. Adenomyosis may involve the uterus focally, creating an adenomyoma, or can be wide-spread within the myometrium. The cause of adenomyosis is unknown, but it has been associated with uterine trauma that disrupts the barrier between the endometrium and myometrium. Such trauma includes that caused by caesarean section or pregnancy termination. Adenomyosis can be diagnosed by transvaginal ultrasound or magnetic resonance imaging.

Treatment options are as for dysmenorrhoea from other causes, namely NSAIDs and hormonal suppression of ovulation for symptomatic relief, with hysterectomy reserved as a last resort option.

ENDOMETRIOSIS

Endometriosis is a condition characterised the presence of ectopic endometrial tissue beyond or outside the uterus. Endometriosis most commonly exists in the lower region of the female pelvis, with the ovaries being involved in approximately half of the cases, and deposits are also commonly found on the broad ligaments, uterosacral ligaments and in the pouch of Douglas. Less commonly, lesions can be found on the bladder, intestines, ureters, and diaphragm (causing severe cyclical shoulder pain); very rarely, endometriosis can be found in distant sites such as the lung, brain, and kidney.

USEFUL WEBSITES

- National Endometriosis Society <www.endo.org.uk>.

- RCOG patient leaflet
  <www.rcog.org.uk/womens-health/clinical-guidance/endometriosis-what-you-need-know>.

Ectopic endometrium acts in the same way as when it is lining the uterine cavity; that is, it grows under the influence of oestrogen during the early proliferative phase of the menstrual cycle, becomes secretory in the second part of the cycle, and desquamates during menstruation. This desquamation and bleeding can cause in intense pelvic and lower back pain during menses. Endometriosis is one of the well-known causes of subfertility.

Diagnosing endometriosis

Laparoscopy is the gold standard investigation used to diagnose endometriosis. Transvaginal ultrasonography and magnetic resonance imaging will demonstrate endometriomata but will not show peritoneal endometriotic deposits.

Medical treatment options for endometriosis

Treatment options for endometriosis are as for dysmenorrhoea due to any other cause; namely, NSAIDs, hormonal suppression of ovulation and, in some cases, 'tricycling' the combined oral contraceptive pill (taking three packets in a row before having 7 days' break). All of these options can be very effective.

Surgical treatment options for endometriosis

Laparoscopy can perform the dual function of diagnosing and treating endometriosis. Laser treatment or surgical excision are the most common ways of removing ectopic endometrial tissue. Hysterectomy, with or without bilateral oophorectomy and salpingectomy, may be performed for extensive disabling disease.

MENSTRUAL PROBLEMS

MENORRHAGIA

During normal menstruation, approximately 40 ml of blood and 35 ml of serous fluid are expelled from the vagina; however, the amount can be extremely variable, both for the same woman on different cycles and between different women. Menorrhagia is the term given for heavy menstrual bleeding and this is a common reason why women go to their GP.

Menorrhagia is an important problem, as it can cause significant inconvenience to the woman; she may require time off work and the bleeding may even confine her to the house as she may require quick and easy access to a toilet. Flooding is the term used for when blood leaks through sanitary towels and clothes, and can be very embarrassing if it occurs in public as the blood can soil clothing and even leak through onto a seat. As a rule of thumb, periods are said to be 'too heavy' when the woman needs to change a large sanitary towel or tampon more than once an hour. Some menorrhagia sufferers may flood despite wearing two tampons and a towel; this is certainly unacceptable and will lead to iron-deficiency anaemia and fatigue if left untreated. There are several options for the management of menorrhagia.

Levonorgestrel-releasing intra-uterine system as a treatment for menorrhagia

The levonorgestrel-releasing intra-uterine system (the Mirena IUS) is currently recommended as the first-line measure in the treatment of menorrhagia, provided that at least 12 months of use is anticipated and the woman does not want to be pregnant. The Mirena IUS delivers progestogen directly to the endometrium, and is highly effective in reducing menstrual bleeding. By 12 months of use, menstrual blood loss is reduced by 95%.

Antifibrinolytic drugs as a treatment for menorrhagia

Tranexamic acid is an antifibrinolytic drug that works by inhibiting plasminogen activator and should be offered as a first-line treatment of menorrhagia in women who do not want a Mirena IUS. Tranexamic acid encourages clot formation within the spiral arterioles and, therefore, reduces menstrual blood loss. Tranexamic acid is taken at a dose of 500 mg tds during menstruation, and can reduce blood loss by 50%. This drug should not be taken by women who are predisposed to thrombo-embolism.

NSAIDs as a treatment for menorrhagia

The non-steroidal anti-inflammatory drug (NSAID) mefenamic acid can be offered as an adjunct drug treatment for heavy menstrual bleeding who also have dysmenorrhoea. It is given at a dose of 500 mg tds during menstruation. It should be taken with food and avoided in those with a history of peptic ulcer.

Combined hormonal contraceptives as a treatment for menorrhagia

Combined hormonal contraceptives (pill, patch or ring) can also be offered as a second-line treatment, depending on the preference and suitability of the individual woman (for young women who have not had a child they may be more acceptable than insertion of an IUS). It must be remembered that both the Mirena IUS and the combined oral contraceptive pill will prevent pregnancy, and so are not be suitable for women who want to conceive.

GOOD PRACTICE POINT 6.4

- Be aware of the contra-indications to combined oral contraceptive methods
  (see Module 7).

Progestogens as a treatment for menorrhagia

The systemic progestogen norethisterone can be taken at the dose of 15 mg od or 5 mg tds from days 5–26 of the menstrual cycle. It is recommended as a third-line measure in the treatment of menorrhagia. The mechanism of action is thought to be by inhibition of ovulation and direct suppression of the endometrium. Although it is not licensed as a contraceptive, it should be avoided by women who want to become pregnant.

In a similar way, injectable progestogens such as depo-provera, can be given as a third-line treatment option.

Endometrial ablation as a treatment for menorrhagia

Endometrial ablation is a surgical technique that can be offered to women in whom medical treatment has failed to control their heavy periods. By ablating (destroying) the full thickness of the endometrium, menstrual flow either ceases completely following treatment, or is greatly reduced. Following treatment, the endometrium cannot accept a fertilised egg for implantation and so this may cause infertility – a significant side-effect. As such, endometrial ablation treatment is not suitable for women who have not completed their family. Pregnancy can be dangerous after endometrial ablation, and an intra-uterine device cannot be safely fitted. Sterilisation is often recommended, otherwise another good contraceptive method is mandatory. Endometrial ablation was discussed in more detail in Module 2.

Surgery as a treatment for menorrhagia

Hysterectomy (surgical removal of the uterus) is reserved for women who have completed their families, and in situations where both medical treatment and endometrial ablation have failed. Hysterectomy is the only treatment option that can guarantee amenorrhoea. If the cause of menorrhagia is uterine fibroids, myomectomy or uterine artery embolisation may be offered rather than hysterectomy in order to retain the woman's fertility.

INTERMENSTRUAL BLEEDING

Bleeding between periods is referred to as intermenstrual bleeding. There are a number of causes for this, and it is important to know and understand these.

Taking a history

As with pelvic pain, the key to helping women complaining of intermenstrual vaginal bleeding is to take a good history of the problem. What is the key factor that has brought the woman to the doctor today, what is her main concern? It is crucial to elicit whether the bleeding is menstrual or intermenstrual. Sometimes, vaginal bleeding occurs during or after sex and this should never be assumed to be normal, and left without investigation.

Menstrual problems

If the vaginal bleeding that is worrying the woman occurs during normal menstruation, she needs re-assurance and education on the menstrual cycle (what to expect and what is normal). Women present to their GP because their periods have 'changed' in some way, perhaps in colour, smell, duration, or perhaps periods are not as regular as they would like. Women can be re-assured that it is normal for periods to be a couple of weeks late at times; as long as pregnancy is excluded, no investigation or treatment is required. Sometimes taking up exercise and achieving a stable sleep pattern makes periods more regular. Stress, anxiety, excessive exercise, weight loss and shift work are all known to delay menstruation. Again, as long as pregnancy is excluded and the cause is clear, the woman can be reassured and attention can be focused on managing the underlying cause (stress management, for example).

Chlamydial/gonococcal infection as a cause of irregular bleeding

Chlamydial infection is an important cause of intermenstrual bleeding and post coital bleeding. Testing for this should be offered in all cases, regardless of sexual history. *Chlamydia* testing is quick and simple as the woman can swab herself in the toilet. It is important to exclude *Chlamydia* before moving on to investigating other causes of bleeding. In areas of high prevalence of gonorrhoea (chiefly inner city areas) gonorrhoea should be sought as well.

Progestogen-only contraceptives as a cause of irregular bleeding

Another common cause of intermenstrual or irregular vaginal bleeding is the use of a progesterone-only contraceptive. Injectable progestogens, the contraceptive implant, the progestogen-only pill, and the Mirena intra-uterine system all cause irregular vaginal bleeding. If one of these contraceptive methods is being used by the woman, this is highly likely to be the cause of her symptoms. As long as she has been tested negative for chlamydia and has an up-to-date smear test, no further investigations are required and the woman can be re-assured.

Some women, although notified of the cause of their irregular bleeding, are unhappy and want something done. There are a number of options:

- The progesterone-only contraceptive can be stopped and an alternative method used, such as the intra-uterine device used.

- If the progesterone-only contraceptive used is the implant, the IUS or an injectable progestogen, the method can be continued and the woman given a 1–3-month trial of the combined oral contraceptive if there are no contra-indications to that, or a progestogen only oral contraceptive if there are contra-indications to the combined pill (Cerazette is the most popular progestogen only oral contraceptive to be used in this way). The usage of oral contraception for this indication is off licence, but it settles the bleeding for the majority of women and subsequent bleeding episodes are often more manageable. Alternatively, mefenamic acid 500 mg bd or tds can be tried.

- If it is the depo-provera causing irregular bleeding and this is occurring 'when the injection is running out', the woman can be invited to have her second injection a week or two early (*i.e.* 10 weeks after the last injection).

- Intermenstrual bleeding at mid-cycle may be related to ovulation. Other causes of intermenstrual bleeding include endometrial and cervical polyps and endometrial cancers.

PROBLEMS CAUSING IRREGULAR MENSTRUATION

POLYCYSTIC OVARIAN SYNDROME (PCOS)

Polycystic ovarian syndrome, known colloquially as PCOS, is a syndrome characterised by hyperandrogenism, hyperinsulinaemia and ovulatory dysfunction. It is a relatively common endocrinopathy, affecting women of reproductive age. The aetiology is unknown, but it is thought that both genetic and environmental factors are responsible for development of the syndrome. There is often a strong family history of PCOS, type II diabetes mellitus, or both of these in sufferers but no clear form of inheritance. It is, therefore, thought that PCOS is a polygenic disorder.

USEFUL WEBSITES

- Verity PCOS Support <www.verity-pcos.org.uk>.

- PCOS Association <www.pcosupport.org>.

- RCOG patient information leaflet <www.rcog.org.uk/womens-health/clinical-guidance/polycystic-ovary-syndrome-what-it-means-your-long-term-health>.

Presentation and symptoms of PCOS

Women with PCOS often complain of irregular or infrequent menstrual periods which is due to infrequent ovulation. Raised androgen levels can result in hirsutism, acne and male pattern alopecia. Most women with PCOS struggle with their weight and many are clinically obese. This is particularly problematic as the increased testosterone production by the excess adipose tissue worsens the symptoms of PCOS further.

The Rotterdam Criteria

The Rotterdam Criteria are agreed diagnostic criteria formulated by the Joint European Society of Human Reproduction an Embryology and the American Society of Reproductive Medicine to diagnose PCOS. According to these criteria PCOS is said to exist if there are at least two out of three of the following signs: (i) oligomenorrhoea or amenorrhoea; (ii) hyperandrogenism; and (iii) polycystic ovaries.

Using these criteria, it is clear that the diagnosis of PCOS is supported by the presence of multiple cysts on the ovaries which give a characteristic appearance when imaged by transvaginal ultrasound scan, but it is possible for a woman to suffer from PCOS even with ovaries that appear normal.

Diagnosing PCOS

Women who present to their GP with irregular or infrequent menstrual periods or hirsutism should be referred for blood tests looking for the presence of PCOS. Typical findings would be:

- Raised serum LH, especially when compared to FSH. The blood sample should be taken between days 2–5 of the menstrual cycle. The higher the LH level the greater the likelihood of anovulation and subfertility.

- Raised serum testosterone; however, many women with PCOS have normal testosterone levels. The testosterone level does not necessarily correlate with the degree of hirsutism or acne.

- Low serum sex hormone binding globulin (SHBG). This is because a lot of the SHBG is bound to testosterone.

- Raised serum prolactin (up to 2000 mU/l).

- All women with PCOS should have a fasting blood sample taken for glucose as impaired glucose tolerance or diabetes mellitus often exists concurrently. If a woman with PCOS falls pregnant, it is important that she is screened for gestational diabetes.

Should the blood test results be suggestive of PCOS, the woman should be referred for transvaginal ultrasound scanning. The diagnosis will be confirmed if the ovaries are found to contain 12 or more follicular cysts, or if the total ovarian volume is greater than 10 cm^3. Transvaginal ultrasound scanning is also helpful as it will identify the presence of ovarian tumours, which may be a potentially fatal cause of virilisation.

Sometimes, an ultrasound scan done for other reasons may show the appearances of polycystic ovaries. If the woman has regular cycles and is symptom free she can be reassured and not treated.

USEFUL WEBSITE

- Long-term consequences of polycystic ovary syndrome (2007)
  <http://www.rcog.org.uk/womens-health/
  clinical-guidance/long-term-consequences-polycystic-ovary-syndrome-green-top-33>.

Treatment of PCOS

Weight loss has been shown to improve insulin sensitivity and to reduce the hyperandrogenaemia associated with PCOS. Therefore all of the symptoms of PCOS are minimised if weight is kept within the ideal range.

The combined oral contraceptive pill is very useful for women with PCOS who do not want to conceive. The oestrogen component increases SHBG and, therefore, decreases circulating androgen levels. The progestogen component suppresses LH secretion. Therefore, a number of symptoms of PCOS are improved when taking a combined pill. Usually a pill such as Dianette is chosen for its anti-androgenic properties.

Although Metformin is not licenced for this indication, it is often given to women with PCOS as it is known to increase insulin sensitivity and decrease serum LH and androgen levels. Metformin, when taken regularly, effectively increases the frequency of ovulation and consequent menstrual periods, and is of benefit to women with PCOS who are trying to conceive.

Anovulatory women who want to conceive can be treated with ovarian stimulants such as Clomiphene in the usual way, as long as they are not obese.

Hirsutism can be treated with limited success with a topical cream such as Vaniqua. Many women try cosmetic treatments such as shaving, waxing or electrolysis in order to remove hairs. but such treatments will need to be funded privately.

MENSTRUAL CESSATION

Menopause

Menopause is an outward sign that the fertility of a woman has come to its close. It is often a very welcome change for those who have experienced years of heavy or painful periods or struggled to control the size of their families using various means of contraception. Conversely, the menopause can be an unwelcome change for women who may feel that their role or ability as a woman has somehow been lessened once they are no longer able to produce progeny. Women may need extra support from their family and friends, as well as healthcare professionals during what can be quite an emotional time.

Perimenopausal symptoms

The period leading up to the menopause is known as the climacteric. There are a number of symptoms a woman may experience during this time, many of which can be slightly uncomfortable or disconcerting.

It is important for a GP to exclude other causes of the woman's symptoms before assuming the perimenopause is the problem. For example, a new prescription of Amlodipine can cause dizziness and hot flushes. Diabetes mellitus, if unrecognised, can cause urinary symptoms and poor concentration. Thyroid disease may cause tremor, tiredness, forgetfulness, dry skin and a dry vagina.

Menstrual changes

The menstrual periods may start to become irregular in frequency, duration, and heaviness. Women may complain that the colour or consistency of their periods is changing.

Hot flushes

Over 80% of women experience hot flushes and/or night sweats during the climacteric period. This is thought to be due to the response of the body to oestrogen withdrawal. Many women will consult their GP about these flushes and sweats as they can be very uncomfortable, embarrassing the woman at work, and disrupting her life quite significantly. They can also disturb sleep resulting in day-time irritability and tiredness. Simple reassurance is often all that is required; however, if hot flushes are frequent and persistent, they may require treatment. In such cases, a trial of evening primrose oil, clonidine, or hormone replacement therapy may be found to be of benefit. Black cohosh is sometimes used, but there have recently been doubts about its safety as it may be hepatotoxic in some women.

Emotional changes

Some women feel that they become more emotionally unstable during this period of their life; for example, they may feel that they cry more easily than they ever did previously. Concentration may be difficult and some women feel that they forget things more often. Whether there is a higher prevalence of depression and anxiety during this time is unclear, but a trial of antidepressants can be given if clear symptoms of depression are being displayed. Scoring using a PHQ-9 questionnaire is recommended good practice to assess and scale depression.

Sexual changes

Women who are perimenopausal or post-menopausal may find that the normal physiological lubricating discharge produced by the vagina is absent. This can cause a feeling of vaginal dryness during the day, and dyspareunia during coitus, especially if there is associated vaginal atrophy. Urinary tract infections may become more frequent. There may also be a loss of libido that may lead to relationship problems if not addressed.

Topical oestrogen creams, pessaries or vaginal rings can greatly improve symptoms of vaginal dryness, dyspareunia, dysuria and urinary frequency. If used regularly there is a need for annual review for any signs or symptoms of endometrial hyperplasia. Hormone-free vaginal moisturisers such as Replens are also often found to be helpful, and are available both on prescription or over-the-counter.

USEFUL WEBSITES

- The British Menopause Society <www.the-bms.org>.

- The Menopause Amarant Trust <www.amarantmenopausetrust.org.uk>.

- The Daisy Network (premature menopause) <www.daisynetwork.org.uk>.

Diagnosing menopause

The menopause is diagnosed in retrospect, after 12 months of secondary amenorrhoea in a woman over the age of 50 years, and after 24 months of secondary amenorrhoea in a woman under the age of 50 years.

Menopause can only be confirmed if the amenorrhoea is not due to an external cause (such as the use of certain ovarian suppressing contraceptives such as depo-provera, anorexia nervosa or malnutrition, etc.).

As a rule of thumb, if a woman is in her late forties or early fifties, and describes typical symptoms such as hot flushes, mood lability, low libido or dry vagina in the months or years before the secondary amenorrhoea, then no investigations are necessary; perimenopause can be diagnosed.

If it has been over 12 months since the last menstrual period, and the woman is over 50 years of age, menopause can be diagnosed and contraception stopped.

If the patient is younger than 44 years of age, then a random FSH test should be performed, followed by a repeated sample a month later. If the serum FSH level is over 20 IU/l, then early peri-menopause can be diagnosed (or early menopause if it has been over 12 months since the last menstrual period).

Premature menopause

Early or premature menopause is said to have occurred if it is reached before the age of 45 years. Menopause can be brought on by radiotherapy or chemotherapy, both of which may induce ovarian failure. Oophorectomy will cause instant menopause. Idiopathic early menopause may run in families.

Early menopause is associated with an increased risk of developing osteoporosis and ischaemic heart disease. For that reason, hormone replacement therapy is recommended until the normal age of menopause has been reached. Note that oestrogens are only cardioprotective in younger post-menopausal women.

A discussion can be had regarding the use of hormone replacement therapy and, if the woman who has reached premature menopause is keen, she should start a cyclical hormone replacement preparation that will bring back cyclical withdrawal bleeds (but not fertility). She can switch to a continuous combined version of HRT, with no bleeding, after a year on the cyclical version.

Postmature menopause

The average age for a woman to reach the menopause in the UK is 52 years. If a woman is still menstruating after the age of 54 years, she should be investigated in order to exclude endometrial malignancy.

HORMONE REPLACEMENT THERAPY

Risks of HRT

Hormone replacement therapy, commonly referred to as HRT, is a very useful treatment for menopausal symptoms. However, HRT carries a small increased risk of developing breast cancer; there are an extra six cases in 1000 for women who use combined HRT for 5 years who are aged between 50–59 years. For the same age group, there will be one extra case in 1000 of stroke in combined HRT users compared to non-users, and 7 extra cases of venous thrombo-embolism. Coronary heart disease risk is confined to older women over the age of 70 years.

There will be 4 extra cases of endometrial cancer in women who use oestrogen-only HRT; for this reason, women with a uterus should always have at least 10 days per cycle of a progestogen added to the oestrogen.

The *BNF* has an HRT risk table which should always be consulted.

Benefits of HRT

HRT lowers the risk of developing osteoporosis in later life if it is used by younger peri- and post-menopausal women. However, HRT should not be given for preventative reasons alone; prescription should be reserved for the alleviation of menopausal symptoms, for which it is extremely effective, and used for as short a time as possible.

Contra-indications to HRT

Contra-indications to HRT include:

- Oestrogen-dependent cancer, history of breast cancer.
- Active thrombophlebitis, active or recent arterial thrombo-embolic disease ,venous thrombo-embolism, or history of recurrent venous thrombo-embolism.
- Liver disease (where liver function tests have failed to return to normal), Dubin–Johnson and Rotor syndromes (or monitor closely).
- Untreated endometrial hyperplasia, undiagnosed vaginal bleeding.

HRT preparations

HRT comes in continuous and cyclical preparations. Continuous preparations are taken continuously (as expected from such a name) and there should be no withdrawal bleeds. Continuous preparations are suitable for women who have already experienced 12 months of secondary amenorrhoea.

Cyclical preparations are also taken continuously, but the colour of the pills or strength of the patches will change as the woman goes through the packet because of changes in the oestrogen and progestogen content. This will result in her having a monthly withdrawal bleed. Cyclical preparations are suitable for women who are perimenopausal and still having periods, or those who have not yet completed 12 full months without a period. Women may consider swapping from a cyclical to continuous preparation once they are over the age of 52 years and withdrawal bleeds are no longer desirable.

HRT comes as oestrogen-only, and combined preparations. Oestrogen-only preparations should be restricted to women who have had a total hysterectomy. For women with a uterus, a combined preparation of oestrogen and progestogen should be used. The progestogen is required to prevent endometrial hyperplasia and the risk of endometrial cancer.

HRT comes as patches, pills and implants. HRT transdermal patches are very popular and work well. They can be stuck onto any part of the skin except on the breasts or over a joint. Patches should be applied to dry skin away from the site of the previous patch in order to reduce the likelihood of developing contact dermatitis. HRT tablets are also popular. A pill is taken daily without a break. The HRT pill cannot be used as an oral contraceptive and this should be made clear to the woman. Oestradiol implants were very popular in the past, but are used less often today. The implants are inserted into the abdominal fascia with the provided trochars every 4–8 months. HRT is also available as a transdermal gel.

Post-menopausal bleeding on HRT

Women on cyclical HRT preparation are expected to bleed every 28 days, and women on a continuous preparation of HRT who have experienced 12 months of amenorrhoea are not expected to bleed at all. A new or changing pattern of bleeding on HRT should be treated in the same way as 'post-menopausal bleeding', that is with tests to exclude the presence of endometrial or cervical cancer. See later in this Module for further details on the management of 'post-menopausal bleeding'.

TIBOLONE

Tibolone is a synthetic steroid with oestrogenic, progestogenic and androgenic actions which is licenced for use in women with menopausal symptoms. It is often found to be particularly helpful in controlling hot flushing. Unlike HRT, it is not associated with increased risk of stroke or breast cancer. However, Tibolone is not often used as it cannot be started in women who have not yet reached 12 months of amenorrhoea (that is in perimenopausal women) as if started then it is associated with unacceptable vaginal bleeding. Tibolone is contra-indicated in women with a history of thrombo-embolism, or ischaemic heart disease.

RALOXIFENE

Raloxifene is a selective oestrogen receptor modulator (SERM) that has been successfully engineered to reduce the incidence of vertebral fractures due to osteoporosis in post-menopausal women. Unfortunately it has not been shown to have any effect in reducing the incidence of hip, neck of femur fractures. However, Raloxifene is also effective in reducing the risk of invasive breast cancer, and has equal efficacy to Tamoxifen (another SERM). Raloxifene does not help menopausal symptoms and should not be prescribed for such, but can be used in post-menopausal women at high risk of developing osteoporosis with the specific aim of minimising vertebral fracture. Raloxifene is, therefore, appropriate for women on long-term corticosteroids, or those with a strong family history of vertebral fracture or spinal degeneration. Raloxifene is taken at a dose of 60 mg daily.

USEFUL REFERENCES

- Vogel VG *et al*. Effects of Tamoxifen vs raloxifene on the risk of developing invasive breast cancer and other disease outcomes: the NSABP Study of Tamoxifen and Raloxifene (STAR) P-2 trial. *JAMA* 2006; **295**: 2727–2741.

- Barrett-Connor E *et al*. Effects of raloxifene on cardiovascular events and breast cancer in postmenopausal women. *N Engl J Med* 2006; **355**: 125–137.

ALTERNATIVES TO PHARMACOLOGICAL HRT

The vast majority of women go through the menopause without requiring any medication or treatment whatsoever. Many women prefer to use herbal remedies to help relieve their symptoms rather than take a prescribed medication, and may ask their doctor for advice about these. On the whole, there is little evidence to support alternative remedies, but many women do find them extremely useful. Smoking cessation, regular exercise and a healthy diet all contribute to a general feeling of well-being.

GOOD PRACTICE POINT 6.5

- Always discuss the alternatives to HRT as well as the different HRT options. Ensure women are well informed on the many choices available to them.

USEFUL WEBSITES

- Patient Information on alternatives to HRT <www.rcog.org.uk/womens-health/clinical-guidance/alternatives-hrt-management-symptoms-menopause>.

- <www.patient.co.uk/health/Menopause-Alternatives-to-HRT.htm>.

POST-MENOPAUSAL BLEEDING

It is never normal to experience vaginal bleeding after menopause has been reached. Should bleeding start, the woman should be examined for any obvious cause, such as a laceration to the vagina caused by traction during intercourse. It is also important to confirm that blood is indeed coming from the vagina and not from the rectum or anus, as it may be difficult for the woman herself to tell. The cervix should be examined and a smear test taken if one is due. Any suspicious lesion on the cervix should be referred immediately for urgent colposcopy, and all other cases of post-menopausal bleeding should be referred to a rapid access clinic. Potential causes of post-menopausal bleeding are discussed below.

Retention of an old intra-uterine device

Some IUDs are inserted and completely forgotten about by the user. If IUD threads are seen, removal should be attempted as this may be the cause of the bleeding. Sometimes, contraction and atrophy of the uterus over an IUD that has been in place for many years can cause difficulty in removal. Such cases can be referred to a gynaecologist or community sexual health clinic for removal.

Endometrial cancer

Should the examination be normal, but symptoms appear genuine, any woman with post-menopausal bleeding should be referred to a rapid-access clinic, where she will be offered a vaginal ultrasound scan to measure the thickness of the endometrium, and an endometrial biopsy. There is no need to wait for the smear test result before referring. Endometrial cancer is discussed in Module 6 and is the most serious cause of post-menopausal bleeding.

Other causes of post-menopausal bleeding include benign polyps and atrophic vaginitis.

UROGYNAECOLOGY

URINARY INCONTINENCE

Urinary incontinence is a common condition affecting many women as well as men, and particularly those of advancing age. It can be defined to be involuntary loss of urine.

USEFUL WEBSITES

- The Continence Foundation <www.continence-foundation.org.uk>.

- The Association for Continence Advice <www.aca.uk.com>.

DETRUSOR INSTABILITY

Detrusor instability, commonly known as 'the unstable bladder' causes symptoms of urinary frequency, urgency, and nocturia. Symptoms may progress to urge incontinence which can be distressing and difficult to manage. The detrusor muscle of the bladder contracts involuntarily.

Treatment for detrusor instability

It is important to make some simple life-style changes in order to manage symptoms of urinary urge incontinence before embarking on pharmacological treatment. It is often helpful if acidic foods (such as citrus fruits) or spicy foods (such as chilli) are avoided as these can irritate the bladder. Some women find that avoiding activities that irritate the urethra such as bathing with bubble bath also helps reduce their symptoms. Alcohol, caffeine and carbonated drinks should be minimised. Some women find it helpful to keep a diary of fluid intake and output, as this can assist in evaluating the problem as well as in monitoring progress once treatment is underway.

It is important that a medication review is done to ensure that the woman is not taking any medications that may exacerbate her urinary symptoms. Drugs that may do so include diuretics, antihistamines, and alpha-blockers.

All women with new incontinence should be checked for the presence of urinary tract infection.

Specialised physiotherapy is often helpful in re-training the bladder. Exercises are taught with the aim of encouraging the bladder to hold larger quantities of urine and to empty fully during urination. It is often helpful to schedule urination at regular intervals throughout the day, and to avoid urination between these times. Kegel exercises, although primarily for women with symptoms of urinary stress incontinence, may be of some benefit to those with detrusor instability symptoms as often the two conditions co-exist.

The most commonly used pharmacological treatments for detrusor instability are anticholinergic agents such as oxybutynin and tolterodine. These are very effective in controlling the symptoms of urge incontinence, but side-effects are common. Side-effects of anticholinergic drugs include dry mouth, and constipation. They are contra-indicated for people with narrow-angle glaucoma.

An alternative treatment for detrusor instability is tricyclic antidepressant drugs such as imipramine or doxepin. Again, treatment is very effective in controlling urge incontinency but side-effects are common, including dry mouth, blurred vision, dizziness and nausea.

STRESS INCONTINENCE

Stress incontinence causes involuntary leakage of urine when coughing, exercising or even stretching. It is due to weak or damaged pelvic floor muscles which result in weakness of the urethral sphincter. Urinary stress incontinence is relatively common after child-birth, and often shows great improvement with pelvic floor exercises.

Surgical treatments for stress incontinence such as insertion of a transvaginal tape are discussed in Module 2, under surgical skills.

USEFUL WEBSITE

- Pelvic Organ Prolapse Information Leaflet
  <www.womenshealthlondon.org.uk/leaflets/prolapse/prolapse.html>.

Pelvic floor exercises

The pelvic floor is a sheet of muscles that extends from the coccyx to the symphysis pubis. It supports the contents of the pelvis and controls the openings of these organs. The pelvic floor also supports the bladder and forms part of the urethral sphincter thus playing a key role in maintaining urinary continence. The pelvic floor surrounds the vagina and provides support for the uterus. The muscles of the vagina play a role in coitus, and help to expel the fetus during childbirth. The pelvic floor also supports the rectum and forms part of the anal sphincter thus maintaining faecal continence (Fig. 6.1).

The muscles of the pelvic floor may be stretched and weakened by child-birth; this can be treated in some part by the woman performing pelvic floor exercises. These exercises basically involve contracting and relaxing the pelvic floor muscles, and can be described to the patient as squeezing below as if 'trying to stop a flow of urine', 'trying to squeeze on a tampon that is falling out' or 'trying to stop yourself from passing wind'. Similar exercises involve inserting weighted devices or 'smart balls' (Fig. 6.2) into the vagina and encouraging the woman to hold

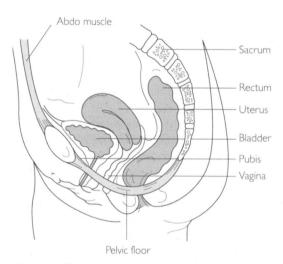

Figure 6.1 The pelvic floor.

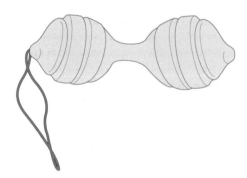

Figure 6.2 'Smart balls' for strengthening the muscles of the pelvic floor.

them in. Such exercises teach the woman how to improve their control over the vaginal wall muscles and pelvic floor muscles, and can strengthen them considerably. This is said to increase both the woman's and her male partner's sexual pleasure (whether post-partum or not) as well as help urinary continence.

SEXUALLY TRANSMITTED INFECTIONS

For management of STIs in pregnancy, see Module 3.

USEFUL WEBSITES

- British Association for Sexual Health and HIV <www.bashh.org>.

- British HIV Association <www.bhiva.org>.

- Chlamydia screening <www.chlamydiascreening.nhs.uk>.

- Condom Essential Wear, STI information for young people <www.condomessentialwear.co.uk/stis-stds>.

Sexuality is central to adult life; sex being a basic requirement of most adults for happiness. Sexual intercourse is the very mechanism of human reproduction and is an essential activity for survival of the species. This has lead to the development of a number of restrictive cultural norms and values to regulate and control sex: with whom, with which gender, with how many different partners, at what age, how frequently, during or not during pregnancy, during or not during menstruation, *etc*.

Most cultures emphasise sexual monogamy through marriage or long-term relationships as key to a functional society. However, ethical and practical norms are often very different, making extra-relationship sex, when it occurs, a secret performance; it is under such conditions that sexually transmitted infections (STIs) are easily transmitted to individuals without their knowledge. Multiple sexual partners also encourage spread of STIs.

In Western society, there has been a sexual revolution occurring since the 1960s, freeing individuals from life-long monogamy and sex only after wedlock. The provision of accessible and effective contraception has lead to the separation of sex from copulation, and sex has increasingly become a pleasurable exercise. The media, advertising, and social factors have lead to a decrease in the age of first sexual experience, and an increase in the average number of sexual partners for both men and women. As a result, there has been a dramatic spread of STIs, although it is unclear whether the prevalence is seemingly higher only because we are screening so much more now (the more people tested the more STIs are found).

Gender is a pivotal fact in personal identity, determining both life experience and options; women are less likely to be able to prevent STI exposure than men. Sexual and economic relationships often limit the freedom of women to negotiate the conditions for sexual intercourse, and there are no widely acceptable female-controlled barrier methods of contraception and STI prevention, (despite the recent development of the female condom). In addition, following exposure to a STI, the female internal anatomy makes women more susceptible to infection and consequent sequelae. Transmission of HIV, gonorrhoea, chlamydia and trichomoniasis are all more efficient from male to female than female to male. This is mainly because there are more bodily fluids transferred from the male to the female during coitus.

Another compounding factor is that women are more likely than men to be asymptomatically infected and, therefore, not seek out treatment. About 50% of women and 10% of men who are infected with gonorrhoea will not have any obvious signs or symptoms. If the woman is symptomatic, there are social stigmas against gynaecological examination in many countries and religions, and social stigmas about a woman having a sexually transmitted infection. This may prevent a woman from seeking diagnosis and treatment. The social stigma attached to STIs is much less for men, and may even be a source of pride.

GOOD PRACTICE POINT 6.6

- Once an STI is found, an HIV test should be considered if not already done.

CHLAMYDIA

Chlamydia is the most common sexually transmitted bacterial infection of humans. Up to 10% of sexually active females under the age of 25 years in the UK who have been tested for *Chlamydia* have been found to be infected. *Chlamydia* is caused by infection with a small, obligate intracellular bacterium called *Chlamydia trachomatis*. Chlamydiae are unusual in that they are unable to synthesize ATP themselves, but rely on a host organism for all of their energy requirements and as a site for replication. They survive extracellularly only as a highly resilient elementary body similar to a spore and it is this form that is responsible for transmission. For *Chlamydia* testing, refer to Module 1.

Symptoms of chlamydia infection

There are often (70% of cases in women) few or no symptoms of chlamydial infection. Therefore, young women (and men) who present to their doctor or sexual health service should always be offered opportunistic screening for genital infection, as they may be unaware of their condition.

Chlamydia can also cause symptoms in many of the infected. Infection of the cervix causes cervicitis. This may present as a purulent cervical or vaginal discharge, dyspareunia, or intermenstrual spotting. Infection of the fallopian tubes causes salpingitis. This may be completely asymptomatic, but leads to infertility if the tubes becomes inflamed and blocked as a result. Infection of the urethra can cause dysuria and urinary frequency issues. In men, chlamydial infection may cause urethral discharge, testicular pain and dysuria.

Treatment of chlamydia

- **First-line** – Azithromycin 1 g stat.

- **Second-line** – Doxycycline 100 mg bd for 7 days

- **In pregnancy** – Erythromycin 500 mg bd for 14 days (azithromycin in pregnancy is off-licence but is used successfully in many genito-urinary clinics in England).

GONORRHOEA

Gonorrhoea is another sexually transmitted infection, common in the UK and world-wide. Gonorrhoea is caused by infection with the Gram-negative diplococcus *Neisseria gonorrhoeae*. *N. gonorrhoeae* dies rapidly in the environment. The only known host is mankind. Like *C. trachomatis*, *N. gonorrhoeae* can colonise mucosal surfaces in the genital tract and cause asymptomatic infections. However, in addition, *N. gonorrhoeae* can pass through mucosal cells and cause inflammation in the underlying tissues. Gonorrhoeal infection may present as a profuse, yellowish-white, vaginal discharge in women, or urethral in men, but it may also be asymptomatic.

Gonorrhoea may infect the rectum in females who receive anal intercourse from an infected male partner, but is generally simply the result of vaginal discharge infecting the rectum. Anal gonorrhoea may be asymptomatic, or may cause rectal discomfort, pain on defecation, and anal discharge. Gonorrhoea in the throat is transmitted by oral sex and is usually asymptomatic.

Treatment of gonorrhoea

The first-line treatment is cefixime 400 mg stat. If allergic to cefixime or penicillin, and for throat infections, use ciprofloxacin 500 mg stat.

Gonorrhoea tends to lose antibiotic sensitivity very rapidly, and so reference to the latest British Association for Sexual Health and HIV (BASHH) guidelines is recommended.

No significant immunity develops to either *N. gonorrhoeae* or *C. trachomatis*, so repeat infection occurs on repeat exposure. Whichever treatment regimen is given, the woman should refrain from sexual activity for 7 days to allow the infection to clear. It is essential that all her sexual contacts are also treated, otherwise she will simply catch the infection again; it should be emphasised that treatment of partners is essential even if no further contact is intended. For women whose partners are known to have gonorrhoea, treatment at the same time as testing is recommended, and also treatment for chlamydia since co-infection occurs in about 40% of women with gonorrhoea and 20% of men. (Note that the reverse is not true, co-infection with gonorrhoea in women with chlamydia is not common).

GOOD PRACTICE POINT 6.7

- Make sure you are up-to-date with current bacterial sensitivities. If you are not sure which antibiotic to give for a STI, contact the on-call microbiologist at your local hospital who can advise. Antibiotic resistance can develop quite quickly in a community so do not assume that last year's choice of antibiotic will be suitable today.

PELVIC INFLAMMATORY DISEASE

When the internal reproductive organs become infected, this is known as pelvic inflammatory disease (PID). *Gardnerella* spp., *N. gonorrhoeae*, *C. trachomatis*, mycoplasma and anaerobes can also occasionally be implicated. Pelvic inflammatory disease can be acute or chronic.

Acute pelvic inflammatory disease

Acute PID is characterised by pelvic pain, vaginal discharge and irregular bleeding. It can make a woman systemically very unwell with fever and malaise. These women often present to accident and emergency departments, as well as to genito-urinary medicine clinics and their GP.

Diagnosis is made by performing a bimanual examination, looking in particular for adnexal tenderness and/or cervical excitation. Microbiological swab tests should be taken for chlamydia and gonorrhoea (see Module 1).

Treatment of pelvic inflammatory disease

Current treatment is with a 14-day course of doxycycline, metronidazole and a stat dose of cefixime (ofloxacin was recommended but, with the increased loss of sensitivity of gonorrhoea to quinolones, it may no longer be appropriate). If the woman is very unwell, she may require hospital admission for intravenous fluids, intravenous ceftriaxone and metronidazole with oral doxycycline. Analgesia should not be forgotten.

Follow-up is recommended at 72 hours and 4 weeks, and partners must be seen, tested, and given a stat dose of Azithromycin as a minimum. Sexual abstinence is needed until treatment and follow-up is complete

Chronic pelvic inflammatory disease

Chronic pelvic infection may go unnoticed, but can lead to long-term pelvic pain and dyspareunia due to inflammation and adhesion formation.

GOOD PRACTICE POINT 6.8

- Pelvic inflammatory disease should be managed as a sexually transmitted infection, but it is not always one and the patient and her partner need to be informed of this.

TRICHOMONAS

Trichomoniasis is another sexually transmitted infection that affects individuals world-wide. It is caused by the single-celled protozoan parasite, *Trichomonas vaginalis*. *T. vaginalis* is able to colonise the vagina and urethra in women, and the urethra in men. It is unique in causing a 'strawberry cervix' in chronically infected women.

Symptoms of trichomoniasis

The typical symptom of infection that women experience is a frothy, yellow-green, vaginal discharge with a strong odour. The infection also may cause dyspareunia and dysuria, as well as irritation and itching of the external genitalia. Most men with trichomoniasis do not have signs or symptoms; however, some develop a urethral irritation or discharge.

Treatment of trichomoniasis

Treatment is with metronidazole 400 mg bd for 5 days (or alternatively 2 g stat). Although the male partner is often asymptomatic, treatment of the male is essential to prevent re-infection of the female partner.

Trichomonas seen on cervical smears

Trichomonas is sometimes reported as present on cervical smear samples. Unfortunately, this has a 30% false-positive rate and so cannot be relied upon. Nonetheless, the result should be discussed with the woman and she may wish either to be treated (as may her partner), or to be investigated further.

GENITAL HERPES

USEFUL WEBSITE

- Herpes virus information <www.herpes.org.uk>.

Genital herpes is a common, sexually transmitted infection that causes recurrent painful genital ulcers in many adults. There is no curative treatment and, as such, genital herpes carries significant morbidity, due to possible breakdown of relationships, psychosexual problems, or depression.

Herpes simplex virus

Genital herpes is caused by the herpes simplex virus, a large double-stranded DNA virus of which there are two types – HSV-I and HSV-II. Both HSV-I and HSV-II can infect the genital area. The prevalence of HSV-II infections in the general population ranges from 10–60%; however, most infections go unrecognised and undiagnosed, simply being carried asymptomatically. Studies consistently show that 90% of people with HSV-II antibodies deny ever having any genital ulceration. However, it is likely that all people who are seropositive for HSV-II antibodies shed HSV-II intermittently. Such 'silent carriers' are infectious to sexual partners.

In developed countries over recent years, the trend of only HSV-II causing genital herpes has changed, and HSV-I now accounts for almost half of new cases. Traditionally, HSV-I was thought only to cause oral cold sores. However, due to increased routine hygiene measures in the home and school there has been a decrease in the exposure of children to HSV-I. Consequently, first contact with HSV-I may not occur until the onset of sexual activity. Previously unexposed young adults do not have immunity to HSV-I, so genital contact results in genital herpes infection. The increasing practice of oral sex clearly contributes to transmission of HSV-I to the genital region.

Symptoms of genital herpes

Individuals with genital herpes suffer from one or more outbreaks of painful, genital ulcers. The severity of symptoms is much greater in individuals with primary genital herpes (the first outbreak), than in subsequent episodes, when established immunity provides some restraint. Genital herpes caused by HSV-II typically recurs four times a year, whereas genital herpes caused by HSV-I typically recurs only once per year.

Genital herpes shares risk factors with other STIs, such as a high number of life-time sexual partners, previous history of STIs, and early age of first sexual intercourse. As with other STIs, women are more susceptible to infection than men.

Treatment of genital herpes

Outbreak duration and severity can be limited by the administration of oral Aciclovir. This is most effective when given as soon as an outbreak occurs, ideally when initial prodromal symptoms of tingling develop. Genital herpes is particularly severe in people with suppressed immune systems, who may suffer from severe outbreaks that are notoriously difficult to control. For any individual who suffers from more than six outbreaks a year, long-term low-dose Aciclovir should be considered, and they are usually best managed in a specialist genito-urinary medicine clinic.

As there is no known antiviral agent that can actually clear the virus, genital herpes can cause significant psychological distress regardless of severity of symptoms. Individuals are infectious to all potential sexual partners and this, in itself, can be highly stigmatising. Use of condoms decreases the risk of transmission considerably, but does not ablate the risk as the herpes simplex virus can be shed from genital and inguinal regions not covered by the condom.

GENITAL WARTS

USEFUL WEBSITES

- BBC Health Information <www.bbc.co.uk/health/conditions/genitalwarts1.shtml>.

- NHS Information <www.nhs.uk/Conditions/Genital_warts/Pages/Introduction.aspx>.

Genital warts are among the most common STI seen at genito-urinary medicine clinics in the UK, and are the most common sexually transmitted viral infection. The incidence of genital wart development is highest among females aged 16–19 years, and in men aged 20–24 years. The warts are unsightly and can be very numerous, but are not painful. Women are more likely to be unaware of their warts than men, as it is more difficult for women to visualise their own genitalia. More commonly, the warts are noticed by their sexual partners.

In women, genital warts usually grow around the introitus, vulva and anus, but can be present on the vaginal walls and cervix as flat warts. Flat warts are not usually visible to the naked eye. Genital warts often grow significantly during pregnancy or with immune suppression. In men, warts develop at the urethral opening, on the glans penis, foreskin, penile shaft, scrotum, and anus.

Human papilloma virus

The human papilloma virus (HPV) is the cause of genital warts. It is a small DNA virus. There are more than 100 different types of HPV, only some of which cause genital warts, other types being responsible for plantar or palmar warts, and cervical cancer. HPV-6 and HPV-11 cause around 90% of cases of genital warts; types 16, 18, 31, 33 and 35 are the cause of warts in the remaining cases.

Treatment of genital warts

First-line treatment is twice daily application of 0.15% podophyllin cream (known as Warticon) to the warts. The recommended regimen is to apply the cream for three consecutive days, then have a 4-day rest. This can be done for up to four consecutive weeks. Podophyllin is a cytotoxic agent and, as such, is contra-indicated in pregnancy and breast feeding.

Should the warts be very large, topical treatment fail, or if topical cytotoxic treatment is contra-indicated, the warts can be removed by cryotherapy (using liquid nitrogen), laser excision, or surgical excision. It should be explained that this treatment is not curative and recurrence is common.

The majority of visible warts are non-oncogenic types and there is no need to increase the frequency of cervical cytology screening if present.

Imiquimod is an immune-response modifier available as a cream. It is not suitable for internal warts or use in pregnancy. It is also extremely expensive, and is best initiated by a genito-urinary specialist.

MOLLUSCUM CONTAGIOSUM

USEFUL WEBSITES

- British Association of Dermatologists information <www.bad.org.uk/site/845/default.aspx>.

- Clinical Knowledge Summary <www.cks.nhs.uk/molluscum_contagiosum>.

- Useful photographs <www.dermis.net/dermisroot/en/13861/diagnose.htm>.

Molluscum contagiosum is a highly contagious skin condition that can be sexually transmitted between adults. It presents as a number of small, pearly-white, non-painful lumps around the groin in males and females. Molluscum contagiosum is also common among children, when it is spread by skin contact or from contaminated towels and flannels, *etc*.

Molluscum is caused by a DNA poxvirus called the molluscum contagiosum virus (MCV), of which there are four types – MCV-1 to MCV-4. MCV-1 is the most prevalent among children, whereas MCV-2 is the most prevalent among adults and is the form that is transmitted most effectively by intimate sexual contact.

Most cases of molluscum self-resolve within 2 years, and there is no need for treatment. If treatment is requested, cryocautery is recommended.

PUBIC LICE

Pubic lice, also known as crab lice, are due to infection by *Pthirsutus pubis*. Lice move by crawling, they can neither hop nor fly. Infestation by pubic lice almost always occurs as a result of intimate sexual contact, but the lice can occasionally be transmitted by physical contact with a contaminated object such as a towel or blanket. Pubic lice are not carried by cats, dogs or any other animal.

P. pubis can be found surviving on coarse hair anywhere on the adult body (axillary hair, chest hair, eyebrows, beard or moustache). However, *P. pubis* is not the usual cause of body lice (caused by *Pediculus humanus corporis*) or head lice (caused by *Pediculus humanus capitis*) and it generally stays within the genital area (Fig. 6.3).

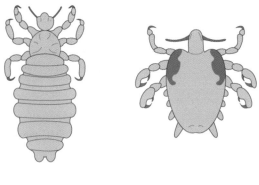

Head louse   Pubic louse

Figure 6.3 Head and pubic lice.

Symptoms and signs of pubic lice

Pubic lice bury their heads in the hair follicles to feed on human blood and, in doing so, cause a local hypersensitivity reaction which results in genital itch. Itching is typically noticed more at night. Although the lice do not cause a rash, repeated scratching can cause the skin to become inflamed and excoriated, and secondary infections such as impetigo may develop. On close examination with a magnifying glass, adult lice of 1–2 mm diameter may be seen on the mons pubis. Small, grey-white, oval egg sacs attached firmly to the base of the hair shaft are often present.

Pubic lice when found on the head or eyelashes of children (where it may cause a blepharitis), although possibly innocent, are a strong indicator of sexual abuse and must be taken seriously.

Treatment of pubic lice

Treatment is by application of 5% Permethrin cream to all body hair. This should be left on for 12 hours before being washed off. A second treatment should occur 3–7 days later. It is advised that all linen and clothing are hot-washed, and that all sexual partners are also treated.

HIV AND AIDS

Infection with the human immunodeficiency virus (HIV) is considered to be the most devastating sexually transmitted infection. Infection with HIV progresses over a number of years to become acquired immunodeficiency syndrome (AIDS) if left untreated. Although AIDS is an extremely distressing illness, HIV is now a treatable medical condition and the majority of those living with the virus remain fit and well on treatment. The importance of screening for HIV is now recognised, but informed consent must be given in a pre-test discussion. Screening in general practice is especially recommended in areas where the local prevalence exceeds 2 in 1000 of the population.

In the UK and other developed nations, progression of HIV infection into AIDS can be prevented in most cases by the daily administration of powerful antiretroviral agents. These medicines are expensive; there are thousands of individuals in developing countries who do not receive treatment and, therefore, die of AIDS. There are parts of sub-Saharan Africa where HIV prevalence among young adults is as high as 33%.

Testing for HIV

The UK national guidelines on HIV testing should be read carefully, note especially the following.

- The list of AIDS-defining conditions (where an HIV test must be offered) includes TB, Kaposi's sarcoma, non-Hodgkin's lymphoma, cervical cancer and cytomegalovirus retinitis (see the guidelines for the full list).

- Many other conditions are listed where HIV testing should be offered, including pregnancy (antenatal or termination clinics), high-grade cervical intra-epithelial neoplasia (CIN) and vaginal intra-epithelial neoplasia, hepatitis B and hepatitis C and indeed any sexually transmitted infection.

- Point of care testing (POCT) is increasingly used; anyone doing these tests should be properly trained in their use. POCT involves screening tests and positives need to be re-tested at a specialist centre. There must be a pathway in place that allows for quick referral.

USEFUL WEBSITE

- UK National Guidelines for HIV Testing <www.bashh.org/guidelines>.

Preconception advice when one partner is HIV positive

If the female partner is HIV positive and the male partner is HIV negative, it is recommended that the woman self-inseminates semen by collecting semen from a used condom, and inserting it high into the vagina using a syringe. This is recommended to protect the uninfected male partner from infection and is usually easily performed by the couple. If the male partner is HIV positive and the female partner is HIV negative, HIV transmission risk per act of unprotected intercourse is reported to be between 0.03–1%. Therefore, sperm-washing is recommended to protect the uninfected female as it is significantly safer than timed unprotected intercourse. However, sperm washing is expensive and currently only provided by a few centres in the UK.

Donor sperm insemination is another option for these couples; however, if this method is used, the genetic material will be from an unknown father, and raises a number of ethical issues.

SYPHILIS

Syphilis is caused by infection with the bacterium *Treponema pallidum*. It is sexually transmitted, but rarely seen in the UK.

First-stage syphilis

A painless ulcer, known as the primary chancre, develops at the site where the bacteria originally entered the body, about a fortnight after exposure. In females, the primary chancre is usually found on the labia, clitoris, or cervix. In males, the primary chancre is typically found on the glans penis, foreskin, or around the anus. The primary chancre is very infectious but, as it is not painful, the ulcer may not be noticed by the individual. Therefore, while the primary chancre is present, and during the second stage, that individual is highly contagious to all sexual partners.

Second-stage syphilis

If first-stage syphilis infection is not treated, the second stage will develop over the following months. Second-stage syphilis has been nick-named 'the great imitator' because so many of the signs and symptoms that occur are indistinguishable from those of other diseases (although these days the same applies to HIV). Such symptoms include:

- A painless rash that is not normally itchy. The rash is typically described as reddish-brown spots on the palms of the hands and soles on the feet. However, it should be remembered that secondary syphilis can cause a rash to appear almost anywhere on the body.

- Condylomata lata lesions are essentially flat, grey, raised lesions that grow on the perineum and vulva of women and around the anus in men. They are easily mistaken for genital warts.

- A flu-like illness with fever, sore throat, malaise, lethargy, and anorexia that can persist for weeks or months. This may be accompanied by a wide-spread lymphadenopathy.

Latent syphilis

The symptoms of secondary syphilis may clear up completely of their own accord, and then *T. pallidum* infection can be carried for years without causing any problems. During this time, the carrier is still infectious to sexual partners.

Third-stage syphilis

If syphilis remains undiscovered and untreated, it may (in about 30% of cases) move into the third stage, some 10–20 years after the infection was contracted. The bacterium damages several organs of the nervous system, cardiovascular system, and of the musculoskeletal system. Signs and symptoms of the late stage of syphilis include poor co-ordination, development of neuropathic joints, gradual onset of blindness, and confusion. As the disease progresses, syphilis causes aortitis, heart failure, paralysis, dementia, and development of the characteristic Argyll–Robertson pupil (the pupil that constricts on accommodation, but not to light). Death is multifactoral.

Treatment of syphilis

An intramuscular injection of penicillin is curative for first- and second-stage syphilis. Penicillin will kill the *T. pallidum* in third-stage syphilis also, but the damage done to end organs will remain. Management of syphilis needs expert experience in a department of genito-urinary medicine, this is especially true for those co-infected with HIV.

CONTACT TRACING

Any individual found to have a sexually transmitted disease should be offered advice and appropriate treatment. A complete sexual history should be taken to ascertain how many sexual partners the individual has had recently, and identify partners who may be infected and require treatment. It is essential that all sexual contacts are contacted and told that they are likely to have an infection. They should be encouraged to attend a sexual health clinic or their GP for diagnostic testing and/or treatment.

All partners who have had unprotected sex with an individual infected with *Chlamydia,* gonorrhoea, non-specific urethritis (NSU) or trichomonas can be offered treatment before their test result comes back, whether or not they are symptomatic.

NON-SEXUAL VAGINAL INFECTIONS

These are not infections in the usual sense but are disturbances of the normal vaginal flora.

VAGINAL CANDIDIASIS (THRUSH)

Candida albicans
Vaginal thrush is a tiresome complaint experienced by most women at least once in their life-time. Thrush is caused by the yeast *Candida albicans*, which can grow in the vagina and/or vulva causing vaginal thrush, or on the mucosa of the tongue, mouth and throat causing oral thrush. *C. albicans* is a yeast that replicates by budding and growing hyphae.

Symptoms and signs of vaginal thrush
Vaginal thrush is characterised by an itchy, vaginal discharge that can be quite uncomfortable. Thrush can be diagnosed by an experienced clinician on examining the vagina, when the typical thick discharge is easily recognised. This discharge is thick and described as of a 'cottage cheese' texture due to the way that the *C. albicans* collects in irregular soft clumps. Sometimes, a thin milky type of discharge may be present. The vulva and vagina may be very sore and red where the hyphae of the organism have broken down the epithelium of the mucosa.

Diagnosing thrush
The diagnosis can be confirmed by taking a charcoal swab, and sending it to a laboratory for microscopy and culture.

Causes of vaginal thrush
Vaginal candidiasis may occur for no apparent reason, but more often is precipitated by antibiotic use (amoxicillin is often causative), or immunosuppression (pregnancy is the main culprit here). Recurrent thrush may also be one of the first signs of diabetes, and there should be a low threshold for at least a urine dipstick test for glucose.

Thrush treatment
Fortunately, treatment for vaginal thrush is easy, cheap, and effective; there is no need to await the results of the swab before offering treatment, indeed treatment for vaginal thrush is available for women to purchase over-the-counter.

Clotrimazole 1% or 2% cream can be applied to the external genitalia two to three times a day until symptoms resolve. In order to combat a vaginal infection, a pessary is needed. This can be placed high into the vagina at bed-time, either with the use of an applicator or a clean finger. The woman should abstain from vaginal sex that night (or use a condom prior to putting in the pessary). If the male partner complains of penile itch, he is welcome to apply clotrimazole cream to the penis, but can be re-assured that his symptoms often resolve without treatment once the female is all clear. It should be emphasised that thrush is not a sexually transmitted infection, and not caused by poor hygiene. Clotrimazole weakens condoms, and patients must be warned about this.

An alternative thrush treatment is an oral tablet of fluconazole 150 mg. This is preferred by some women, particularly those who do not like to feel inside their vagina. Fluconazole should be used with caution in those with liver problems, and avoided completely during pregnancy and breast feeding.

BACTERIAL VAGINOSIS

Bacterial vaginosis is another troublesome, common complaint of a great many women. It affects almost one-third of sexually active women at some point during their life. Bacterial vaginosis occurs in susceptible women when they wash inside the vagina with soap, use fragranced feminine hygiene products, genital perfumes or scented bubble baths. It presents as an offensive vaginal discharge which is characteristically described as being 'fishy'. The smell is particularly prominent during, and just after, coitus, which can be extremely embarrassing. This is due to semen being alkaline. The smell may also be more noticeable following a menstrual period. The more the woman washes and douches the vagina with soap, the more pungent the smell will become.

Another problem is that bacterial vaginosis in the third trimester of pregnancy can lead to the onset of premature labour especially in those who have already had a premature birth.

Cause of bacterial vaginosis

Bacterial vaginosis is due to the overgrowth of normal vaginal commensal organisms, particularly anaerobes, rather than being an infection due to one particular organism. Common culprits are *Gardnerella* spp., *Escherichia coli*, *Bacteroides* spp. and *Mobiluncus* spp. Bacterial vaginosis is not sexually transmitted and does not affect the male partner in any way.

Diagnosing bacterial vaginosis

The history itself is often quite indicative of bacterial vaginosis; however, it is always prudent to examine a woman to be sure. The odour of bacterial vaginosis is quite easily recognised by doctors and nurses when performing a speculum examination but, if the diagnosis is in doubt, some vaginal discharge can be put on a strip of litmus paper and the pH tested. An alkaline pH (over pH 7) is highly suggestive of bacterial vaginosis. A charcoal swab can be taken from the high vagina and sent to the laboratory for microscopy. Clue cells are an indication of bacterial vaginosis; however, clue cells are found in one-fifth of all women who have charcoal swabs taken and many do not complain of any of the symptoms of bacterial vaginosis. Clue cells are squamous epithelial cells with their borders obscured by innumerable tiny coccobacilli. If these are seen on microscopy, but the woman is asymptomatic, no treatment is required. However, if the woman is symptomatic and clue cells are present, this can be taken as a diagnosis of bacterial vaginosis.

Bacterial vaginosis treatment

Treatment is with a 5-day course of metronidazole 400 mg bd. It is essential to avoid alcohol during treatment as it causes a disulfiram-like reaction and can occasionally make the woman collapse. An alternative treatment regimen is to insert an applicator full of clindamycin 2% vaginal cream into the vagina each night for seven nights, or to insert an applicator full of metronidazole 0.75% vaginal gel into the vagina each night for five nights. The woman must be made aware that these vaginal treatments may damage condoms.

Recurrent bacterial vaginosis is common; if the woman knows the symptoms well and sexually transmitted infections are excluded, there is no need to carry out repeated swabs for each episode. It is reasonable to provide treatment on request.

GOOD PRACTICE POINT 6.9

- The avoidance of excessive washing, antiseptics and 'feminine hygiene products' is at least as important as antibiotics in treating bacterial vaginosis.

NON-INFECTIOUS VULVO-VAGINAL CONDITIONS

It is always advisable to do a speculum examination the first time a women gets a vaginal discharge. Retained tampons, bits of broken condoms, forgotten diaphragms, and more exotic objects may be found, as may a serious pathology such as a cervical carcinoma.

LICHEN SCLEROSUS

> ### USEFUL WEBSITES
>
> - British Association Dermatologists Lichen Sclerosus Guideline
>   <www.bad.org.uk/Portals/_Bad/Guidelines/Clinical%20Guidelines/Lichen%20Sclerosus.pdf>.
>
> - Lichen Sclerosus BBC Health Information
>   <www.bbc.co.uk/health/conditions/lichensclerosus1.shtml>.
>
> - National Lichen Sclerosus Support Group <www.lichensclerosus.org/>.

Lichen sclerosus is a chronic inflammatory skin disease that causes substantial discomfort and morbidity, most commonly in adult women, but also children. Typically, lichen sclerosis affects older women, who have already achieved the menopause. Any skin site may be affected including, rarely, the oral mucosa, but lichen sclerosus is most common in the anogenital area where it predisposes to the development of vulval cancer.

Symptoms and signs of lichen sclerosus

Lichen sclerosus is a cause of intractable itching and soreness, which can lead to extensive scar formation. In children, it can be difficult to differentiate the disorder from changes that can be caused by sexual abuse, and this has led to many upsets. In such cases, it may be best to involve a dermatologist (who can take a biopsy of the lesions) or paediatrician (who is experienced in the behaviour of children who are suffering from abuse).

Some women who suffer from lichen sclerosus experience pain on urination and defecation, and may develop recurrent anal fissures. Superficial dyspareunia is common, with painful tears occurring with sexual intercourse. Other patients have no symptoms at all, and the condition is simply picked up on routine examination of the external genitalia.

The typical appearance of lichen sclerosus is a hyperkeratotic patch of pale white skin between the labia majora. It may be localised to one small area and can be very itchy. Scarring may distort the skin texture, causing a loss of the normal labial folds, closure of the labia majora over the clitoris, or narrowing of the vaginal introitus.

Cause of lichen sclerosus

The underlying cause of lichen sclerosus is unknown, but there seems to be a genetic susceptibility to development of the condition and a link with other autoimmune diseases. The Koebner phenomenon is known to occur (i.e. the lesions of lichen sclerosus may occur at areas of previously traumatised skin), so trauma, injury, and sexual abuse have been suggested as possible triggers of symptoms in genetically predisposed people.

Treatment of lichen sclerosus

Unfortunately, there is no cure for lichen sclerosus, but the application of a potent topical corticosteroid ointment such as betamethasone gives good symptomatic benefit. Lignocaine gel may be applied to the vulva before sex to numb the area, thus allowing non-painful penetration of the penis. Women with lichen sclerosus should be reviewed regularly because of the small risk of malignant change.

EARLY PREGNANCY PROBLEMS

ECTOPIC PREGNANCY

USEFUL WEBSITES

- The Ectopic Pregnancy Trust <www.ectopic.org.uk/>.

- The Ectopic Pregnancy Foundation <www.ectopicpregnancy.co.uk/>.

An ectopic pregnancy is one in which the fertilised ovum is implanted in a tissue other than the endometrial lining of the uterus. It occurs in approximately 1% of pregnancies. Most ectopic pregnancies occur within one or other of the fallopian tubes, but implantation can also occur in the cervix, ovaries, or abdomen.

Risk factors for the development of an ectopic pregnancy are:

- Any tubal pathology.

- Previous ectopic pregnancy.

- Previous pelvic inflammatory disease.

- Previous chlamydia infection.

- Previous pelvic surgery, including tubal surgery/sterilisation.

- Smoking.

- Advanced maternal age.

- A failed intra-uterine contraceptive device or failed tubal ligation.

Pregnancy is rare when an intra-uterine contraceptive device (IUCD) is *in situ*, or when the fallopian tubes have been clipped or cauterised as part of a sterilisation procedure. The quoted failure rate when consenting a patient for a laparoscopic clip sterilisation is 1 in 200. Should the IUCD or tubal ligation fail, approximately one in five of those pregnancies will be ectopic. It should be made clear that the overall risk of ectopic pregnancy in women using the IUCD or sterilisation is much lower than women not using a contraceptive method.

If left untreated, about half of ectopic pregnancies will resolve naturally; the implanting embryo burrows actively into the tubal lining, and invades vessels causing bleeding. This intratubal bleeding (haematosalpinx) expels the implantation out of the fallopian tube as a spontaneous tubal abortion. The rest of the ectopic pregnancies may succeed in implantation. In these cases, the embryo can grow and develop within the fallopian tube or other ectopic site. Prostaglandin release by the stretched tube will cause deep iliac fossa pain, and attachment of the placental villae into the lining of the tube may cause some vaginal bleeding. Untreated, the pregnancy may rupture through the wall of the fallopian tube into the abdomen causing an intraperitoneal haemorrhage that can be fatal.

In the last triennial report from CEMACH covering maternal deaths in the UK in 2005–2008, there were 10 deaths from ectopic pregnancies in the UK.

Ectopic pregnancy may be suspected on history taking, and any woman complaining of pelvic pain within the first trimester of pregnancy should be sent for a transvaginal ultrasound scan to determine whether her pregnancy is intra-uterine or ectopic. Most ectopic pregnancies present between 6–8 weeks after the last menstrual period. Some present before the woman knows that she is pregnant, so all women of reproductive age complaining of pelvic pain should have a pregnancy test.

Medical treatment of ectopic pregnancy

Early treatment of an ectopic pregnancy with the antimetabolite methotrexate has proven to be very effective, and is now often first-line treatment for women who are haemodynamically stable, with a serum hCG below 4000 IU/l, an ectopic pregnancy measuring less than 3 cm, and minimal symptoms.

The woman must be admitted to hospital for administration of the methotrexate to allow her condition to be monitored safely. Methotrexate is given as a single intramuscular dose, calculated according to the woman's weight, and must be administered with great care (wear gloves to draw up the medicine) by a doctor who is neither pregnant nor trying for a pregnancy. The death of the ectopic pregnancy is then monitored by transvaginal ultrasound scanning and serial serum hCG measurements. Some women may require a second dose of methotrexate.

Women should be advised to avoid sexual intercourse during treatment, to maintain ample fluid intake and to use reliable contraception until treatment is complete and she is discharged from follow-up. This is because there is a clear teratogenic risk to future pregnancies while methotrexate remains in the mother's system.

Surgical treatment of ectopic pregnancy

Surgical intervention is required for women with a high serum hCG concentration at presentation; methotrexate treatment is likely to fail with levels of serum hCG over 4000 IU/l. The presence of cardiac activity in an ectopic pregnancy means that methotrexate treatment will be contra-indicated and early surgical intervention will be required. Urgent surgery will be required if the woman is showing any signs of shock and if the ectopic pregnancy has already ruptured.

The surgeon can choose to carry out a salpingostomy (removal of the pregnancy with conservation of the fallopian tube) or salpingectomy (removal of the fallopian tube with the pregnancy). This is a difficult decision to make and will depend on the experience and skill of the surgeon, and the condition of the fallopian tube. Tube preservation is preferred if possible, in order to maximise future fertility. Infertility occurs in many women who have had an ectopic pregnancy but, according to data from the Ectopic Pregnancy Trust, 65% of women overall will becomes pregnant again within 18 months of having an ectopic pregnancy.

Laparoscopic surgery is preferred to open laparotomy as laparoscopic procedures are associated with shorter operation times, less intra-operative blood loss, shorter hospital stays and lower analgesic requirements. However, if the ectopic pregnancy has ruptured and a haemoperitoneum has developed, urgent laparotomy may be required to stop the bleeding as quickly as possible, and save the woman's life.

Expectant management of pregnancy of unknown location

All intra-uterine pregnancies with a serum hCG level of approximately 1000 IU/l – sometimes referred to as the discriminatory level – should be clearly visible on transvaginal ultrasound scanning. When serum hCG levels are below 1000 IU/l and there is no pregnancy (intra- or extra-uterine) visible on transvaginal ultrasound scan, the pregnancy can be described as being 'of unknown location', and may well be a pregnancy (intra- or extra-uterine) that is spontaneously resolving. Low initial hCG levels are a significant predictor of spontaneous resolution.

Using an initial upper level of serum hCG of 1000–1500 IU/l to diagnose pregnancy of unknown location, women with minimal or no symptoms of ectopic pregnancy, and no blood in the pouch of Douglas, can be safely managed expectantly with twice weekly serum hCG measurements and weekly transvaginal scans until hCG levels are less than 20 IU/l. Such women should be considered for active intervention if symptoms of ectopic pregnancy occur, or serum hCG levels rise above the discriminatory level.

MISCARRIAGE

Miscarriage is the spontaneous loss of pregnancy prior to 24 weeks' gestation. Miscarriage is very common, with up to one-third of conceptions being lost within the first 6 weeks of gestation (this figure is high as it includes an estimate of the conceptions that do not even reach the stage of implantation). The incidence of miscarriage decreases as the pregnancy develops, and occurs in approximately 15% of clinically confirmed pregnancies within the first 12 weeks of gestation, and 2% of pregnancies of over 14 weeks' gestation.

The likelihood of miscarriage increases with increased maternal age; a 40-year-old woman is twice as likely to miscarry as a 20-year-old. This is probably due to the increased incidence of fetal genetic abnormalities in older mothers.

Early miscarriage goes unrecognised in many cases, being interpreted by the woman as being a late, heavy period.

USEFUL WEBSITES

- The Miscarriage Association <www.miscarriageassociation.org.uk/>.

- Miscarriage Support (Scotland) <www.miscarriagesupport.org.uk/>.

- Stillbirth & Neonatal Death Society SANDS <www.uk-sands.org/>.

Recurrent miscarriage

Miscarriage is so common that routine investigation for a maternal cause is not required for one or two events. Miscarriage in most cases represents the natural loss of a non-viable fetus, and the majority of women go on to have successful pregnancies following a miscarriage. However, if a woman suffers three or more miscarriages in a row, this is defined as recurrent miscarriage and there may be an underlying abnormality predisposing to poor pregnancy outcome.

Maternal causes of recurrent miscarriage include antiphospholipid syndrome and thrombophilias such as protein C deficiency, protein S deficiency and antithrombin III deficiency. Once diagnosed, the woman should be treated with low-dose aspirin throughout a subsequent pregnancy. Women with antiphospholipid syndrome should also be treated throughout the pregnancy with low molecular weight heparin once their pregnancy has been confirmed and a fetal heart seen on a scan.

Uterine abnormalities are the cause of recurrent miscarriage in some cases. Such abnormalities include fibroids that distort the uterine cavity and congenital uterine abnormalities, such as a bicornate uterus.

Rarely, recurrent miscarriage can be due to one or both partners having an abnormal karyotype such as a balanced translocation. These patients need advice from a genetics specialist.

However, for most women who suffer recurrent miscarriage, there is no cause found.

Classification of miscarriage

There is alternate terminology used for different types of miscarriage.

- **Threatened miscarriage** – the term given to vaginal bleeding in early pregnancy with a closed cervix. In such cases, a miscarriage may occur or bleeding may spontaneously resolve as the pregnancy continues. The fetal heart beat should be visible on transvaginal ultrasound scanning.

- **Inevitable miscarriage** – the term given to vaginal bleeding in early pregnancy with an open cervix. The woman may experience vaginal bleeding with the passage of clots and tissue. There is often accompanying cramping pelvic pain. In such instances, it is just a matter of time before the products of conception are expelled from the uterus.

- **Incomplete miscarriage** – the term used when some products of conception have been expelled from the uterus, but some remain inside. This is identified on transvaginal ultrasound scanning, but will be apparent on clinical examination because the uterus will feel bulky and tender.

- **Complete miscarriage** – the term used when all products of conception have been expelled from the uterus.

- **Missed miscarriage** – the term used when the fetus has died, but the products of conception remain in the uterus. There may not have been any untoward signs detected by the mother, and so missed miscarriage may be an unexpected finding on routine ultrasound scanning when no fetal heart beat can be found.

Management of miscarriage

Many women who experience pelvic pain or vaginal bleeding during early pregnancy are concerned, as they know pain and bleeding are signs that they may be losing their pregnancy. It is important for the doctor to acknowledge their fears, and to try to be re-assuring if this is appropriate.

An assessment must be made to determine whether miscarriage is threatened, inevitable, incomplete or complete. This is done by speculum examination to see whether or not the cervix has dilated, and by transvaginal ultrasound scanning.

When a miscarriage is threatened, the woman can be treated supportively with weekly ultrasound monitoring. When a miscarriage is inevitable and the bleeding is light, the woman can be reviewed in 2 weeks' time and re-scanned. On re-scan, if there are retained products of conception, she can be given oral misoprostol to induce cervical dilatation and uterine contractions to expel the pregnancy. Alternatively, surgical evacuation of retained products of conception (ERPC) can be offered, which is also the advised treatment if bleeding is heavy or prolonged. When the miscarriage is incomplete and products of conception are seen passing through an open cervix, these can be pulled out gently using Spencer Wells or sponge-holding forceps.

In all cases, anti-D must be administered if the woman is Rhesus negative.

MOLAR PREGNANCY

Hydatidiform moles are a result of non-viable conceptions. Every cell of a complete hydatidiform mole is paternal in origin; there is no genetic information from the mother. This is most often due to dispermic fertilisation of an anucleate ovum, but there are other errors of fertilisation that can result in this genotype. A molar pregnancy affects one in 700–800 pregnancies in the UK. Of interest, one in ten hydatidiform moles is accompanied by a co-existing fetus and is referred to as a partial mole.

USEFUL WEBSITE

- Charing Cross Hospital Hydatiform Mole and Choriocarcinoma Support Service
  <www.hmole-chorio.org.uk/patients_info_intro.html>.

Development of the blastocyst

Fertilisation of the ovum by the sperm occurs in the fallopian tubes. The fertilised egg is carried down to the uterus by muscular contractions of the fallopian tubes and movement of cilia. By the time the embryo reaches the uterine lumen, it has divided many times to become a ball of cells known as the blastocyst. The blastocyst consists of two distinctive cell groups: the embryoblast or inner cell mass which will become the embryo, and the trophoblast which will become the placenta. The centre of the blastocyst is fluid filled (Fig. 6.4).

Implantation

When the blastocyst comes into contact with the endometrial epithelium, degradative proteases are released by the trophoblast which results in the trophoblast sticking to the endometrium. Implantation of the blastocyst occurs as the trophoblast erodes deep into the endometrium. Numerous villi grow which have a high surface area to volume ratio to facilitate gas exchange and nutrient transfer.

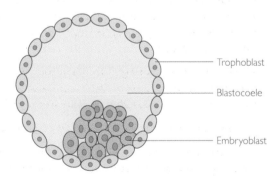

Figure 6.4 The blastocyst.

In the case of a molar pregnancy, the blastocyst does not grow as a normal conception would. Instead there is gross proliferation of the trophoblast. This results in the blastocyst developing into a hydatidiform mole rather than a fetus and placenta.

Carcinogenic potential of a molar pregnancy

Hydatidiform moles are characterised by premalignant expansive growth and have carcinogenic potential; between 8–20% of complete molar pregnancies result in neoplasia.

Predisposing factors to molar pregnancy

Hydatidiform moles affect women throughout the reproductive age range but are more common at the extremes of age. Women under the age of 16 years have a six times higher risk of developing the disease than those aged 16–40 years, and women who conceive aged 50 years or more have a one in three chance of having a molar pregnancy.

There is a higher incidence of molar pregnancy among Far Eastern women. The reason for this is unclear.

Presentation of a woman with molar pregnancy

A patient with a molar pregnancy may present with vaginal bleeding in early pregnancy, or exaggerated symptoms of pregnancy. However, in most cases, molar pregnancies are asymptomatic and are picked up on routine antenatal ultrasound scanning. Diagnosis can be confirmed by raised levels of serum hCG, which is secreted in abnormally large quantities by the proliferating trophoblast.

Treatment of molar pregnancy

If left untreated, a hydatidiform mole will almost always end as a spontaneous abortion. However, the potential risks of this condition are too dangerous to allow the pregnancy to continue and so termination of pregnancy is recommended.

Following molar pregnancy termination

Because of the risk of malignancy, there is a clear need for rigorous surveillance of women following termination of their molar pregnancy. All women with trophoblastic disease are, therefore, registered for follow-up with a specialist centre such as Charing Cross Hospital.

Follow-up involves blood tests for serum hCG, the level of which should return to normal within 8 weeks and stay low. The woman is advised not become pregnant again for at least 6 months after the termination to allow for monitoring. However, the use of hormonal methods may be linked to an increased risk of neoplastic change, and intra-uterine devices should not be fitted if the hCG is still high. Therefore, barrier methods are recommended, which may be difficult for some women. Should hCG start to rise (and the woman is not carrying a new pregnancy), or should hCG remain greater than 20,000 IU/l more than 4 weeks after termination of pregnancy, chemotherapy is needed. If choriocarcinoma is recognised and treated early, it has a very good prognosis, with cure rates of 95%.

ANEMBRYONIC PREGNANCY

Anembryonic pregnancy occurs when the embryo suffers an early death and is re-absorbed, leaving an empty gestation sac in the uterus. Again, this may be picked up unexpectedly on a routine ultrasound scan.

GYNAECOLOGICAL CANCERS

CERVICAL CANCER

The annual incidence of cervical cancer in the UK is 9.7 per 100,000 women, with a mortality rate of 3.7 per 100,000 women. Squamous cell cervical carcinoma is caused by sexually transmitted infection with human papilloma virus; over 99% of cervical cancers are positive for either HPV-16 or HPV-18.

Risk factors for development of cervical cancer

Because cervical cancer is a result of a sexually transmitted infection, it is more likely to develop in women who started sexual activity at a young age, and those who have had unprotected sex with multiple partners. Cigarette smoking is an additional risk factor for the development of cervical cancer; this is thought to be because smoking reduces the immunity of the cervical mucosa to HPV infection. The combined oral contraceptive pill is associated with cervical cancer, but it is thought that this is incidental rather than causal, and should not deter women with HPV from using the combined pill.

Anatomy of the cervix

The cervix is the narrower more cylindrical lower portion of the uterus. It is made up of the ectocervix (outside part), and endocervix (inside part). The ectocervix is the portion of the cervix easily visible on speculum examination (Fig. 6.5).

The ectocervix is covered by a pink, stratified, squamous epithelium, and is suitable for the hostile life at the top of the vagina, which includes contact with the penis during coitus. The endocervix lies within the cervical canal, out of sight. It is covered by a reddish columnar epithelium consisting of a single layer of cells and is rather more delicate than the ectocervix.

The area where the squamous epithelium meets the columnar epithelium is known as the transformation zone. Before puberty, the transformation zone lies within the cervical canal and cannot be seen. After puberty, the columnar epithelium extends onto the ectocervix and can often be seen on speculum examination. Almost all cervical cancers occur in the transformation zone, so it is from this region that cells are harvested for cervical screening, and it is identification of this area that is of great importance in colposcopy.

Ectropion refers to more pronounced eversion of the columnar epithelium onto the ectocervix than is usual. This occurs under the influence of extra oestrogen, such as when taking the combined oral contraceptive pill, or during pregnancy.

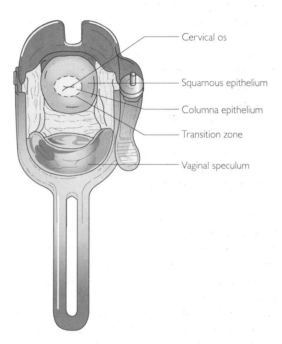

Figure 6.5 View of the ectocervix through the Cusco speculum.

Cervical intra-epithelial neoplasia

Cervical intra-epithelial neoplasia (CIN) is the histological term used to describe precancerous changes seen in the epithelial cells that are harvested by cervical screening. CIN-I is equivalent to mild dysplasia, CIN-II to moderate dysplasia, and CIN-III to severe dysplasia, or carcinoma *in situ*.

Symptoms and signs of cervical cancer

Cervical cancer has no symptoms until it is quite advanced, having passed through the precancerous stages of CIN-I, CIN-II and CIN-III. Once at the invasive stage, cervical cancer presents with intermenstrual or post-coital bleeding, menorrhagia, or an offensive vaginal discharge. Advanced, late-stage disease causes malaise, weight loss and an iron-deficiency anaemia.

On speculum examination, an ulcerated lesion or mass may be seen on the cervix, which often bleeds when touched. Such cases need rapid referral to a gynaecological oncologist.

Metastatic cervical cancer

Cervical cancer spreads directly through the uterus, vagina, bladder or rectum to cause fistulae. Cervical cancer can also spread indirectly via the lymphatic system to metastasise throughout the pelvis. Treatment is with chemotherapy and radiotherapy.

THE CERVICAL SCREENING PROGRAMME

As precancerous cervical cells cause no symptoms, they can only be detected by a screening method. The NHS Cervical Screening Programme was introduced in 1987 to detect women with precancerous cervical cells before they progress to invasive cervical cancer. The NHS Cervical Screening Programme in England and Northern Ireland invites women for a 'smear test' every 3–5 years between the ages of 25–65 years (ages of 20–64 years for Wales, 20–60 years for Scotland).

Only women who have been sexually active require the test (note women who have sex with women should be included). A total of four million tests are done annually in the UK. Cervical screening is carried out by GPs, practice nurses, sexual health clinics, and at colposcopy. Cervical screening is also offered privately by a number of well-woman clinics.

USEFUL WEBSITES

- Patient information on cervical cancer <www.cancerhelp.org.uk>.

- Department of Health information on cervical screening <www.cancerscreening.nhs.uk/cervical/index.html>.

- Patient information leaflet on colposcopy <www.cks.nhs.uk/patient_information_leaflet/colposcopy>.

- HPV vaccine information <www.immunisation.nhs.uk/Vaccines/HPV>.

The 'smear test'

Papanicolaou's technique (known as the Pap smear) of smearing exfoliated cervical cells onto a slide and examination under a microscope has been used world-wide as a means of preventing cervical cancer since the 1940s. The test has remained virtually unchanged to the present day, only recently being superseded by liquid-based cytology.

Liquid-based cytology

Liquid-based cytology is a new way of preparing cervical samples for examination; it has now replaced the Pap smear test in almost all areas. Cells are collected from the cervix using a brush and then washed into a vial of preservative fluid. In the laboratory, cellular debris such as blood or mucus is removed, and the cervical cells examined under a microscope.

Cervical screening results

In the UK, screening results are categorised using the British Society of Clinical Cytologists (BSCC) guidelines depending on the degree of dyskaryosis as negative, borderline, mild, moderate, severe or inadequate.

Inadequate results

Common causes of inadequate smears include contamination of the sample with lubricant (used to ease insertion of the speculum), contamination of the sample with polymorph infiltrate (from the thick mucus plug in the cervical os), and scanty collection (not enough cells picked up on the brush).

Inadequate smears can be a source of significant distress to women, and a waste of resources in general practices, clinics and cytology laboratories, as the test needs to be repeated. By not using any lubricant on the speculum and removing the mucus plug from the os with a damp swab before taking the sample, the inadequate rate is greatly reduced.

GOOD PRACTICE POINT 6.10

- Remember not to use lubricant on the speculum when taking cervical cytology as it can lead to inadequate results.

Borderline and mild dyskaryosis

A borderline result is given when there are nuclear changes seen which cannot be regarded as normal, but it is not clear whether they actually represent cellular abnormality or not. The majority of such changes revert back to normal within 6 months when the woman should be re-tested.

The result 'mild dyskaryosis' indicates that nuclear changes were seen. As with borderline results, the majority of such changes revert back to normal within 6 months. Two consecutive samples showing mild dyskaryosis indicate colposcopy referral.

Moderate and severe dyskaryosis

Moderate and severe dyskaryosis both require colposcopic examination and likely treatment.

Invasive cancer

Very occasionally, invasive cancer or glandular neoplasia may be reported from a cervical screening test. Such a patient requires urgent referral to a gynaecological oncologist.

COLPOSCOPY

Colposcopy is the visual examination of the cervix using a binocular microscope, known as a colposcope. Colposcopy can be offered in the community or hospital setting. Acetic acid solution and/or iodine solution are applied to the cervix to improve visualisation of the transformation zone.

HPV VACCINATION

Routine HPV vaccination was introduced for all girls in the UK aged 12–13 years as part of the national immunisation programme in September 2008. The programme is delivered through secondary schools, and consists of three injections given over a 6-month period. A catch-up campaign is offered to girls through schools who are between 13–18 years of age; however, to provide the most benefit and protection, the vaccine needs to be given before any sexual activity begins. Women above the age of 18 years can request the vaccine from their practice nurse if they have not yet had penetrative sex.

The HPV vaccine has been shown to be effective for 4.5 years after completing the course. Beyond that, it is not known how long the vaccine protection lasts.

Ethical debate around HPV vaccination

The notion that vaccinating against a sexually transmitted infection might encourage risky sexual behaviour has received media and academic interest, and some parents (more so in the USA than in the UK) have refused consent for their daughter to participate in the school vaccination programme on this basis. Those 12–16-year-old girls whose parents refuse consent to participate in the school vaccination programme and are assessed to be 'Fraser competent' have access to the vaccine from their GP or practice nurse.

Cervarix versus Gardasil

HPV-16 and HPV-18 together cause over 70% of squamous cell cancers. HPV-18 alone causes around 50% of all adenocarcinomas. Cervarix is a bivalent vaccine that provides protection against HPV-16 and HPV-18, and is the vaccine used for the NHS vaccination programme.

The quadravalent HPV vaccine Gardasil provides protection against HPV-11 and HPV-6 in addition to HPV-16 and HPV-18, and so decreases the likelihood of developing genital warts as well as cervical cancer in sexually active females.

BREAST CANCER

USEFUL WEBSITES

- Breakthrough Breast Cancer <http://breakthrough.org.uk/breast_cancer/>.

- Breast Cancer Awareness <www.cancerresearchuk.org/breastcancer>.

- Breast Cancer Care <www.breastcancercare.org.uk/>.

- *NICE Guidance Early & Locally Advanced Breast Cancer* <http://guidance.nice.org.uk/CG80 >.

- *NICE Guidance Familial Breast Cancer* <http://www.nice.org.uk/CG014>.

Breast cancer is extremely rare before the age of 25 years. It then increases in incidence steadily with increasing age. In developed countries, one woman in ten will develop breast cancer, and one in eighteen will die from it.

The first symptom of breast cancer is usually a new lump in the breast, found by the woman or her partner. Sinister features of a lump, that give an indication that the lump may be cancerous, include changes in breast size or shape, skin dimpling, nipple inversion, and nipple discharge. Infiltration of the carcinoma into the overlying skin results in skin oedema with a characteristic dimpling of the skin known as 'peau d'orange' (like orange peel). Pain is a very non-specific symptom and, although is present in approximately 10% of breast lumps, may also be due to a number of completely benign causes.

Common sites of metastasis include bone, liver, lung and brain.

Breast cancer screening

Breast cancer screening is an attempt to identify breast cancers at an early stage, before they have become symptomatic, and when curative treatment is still possible. The screening methods used in the UK are encouragement of self-examination, X-ray mammography, and breast magnetic resonance imaging (MRI). Genetic testing is offered to women with a strong family history of breast cancer in first-degree relatives.

Breast self-examination

Breast self-examination can be taught by a trained healthcare professional or self-taught from books, television or the internet. Examination involves the woman systematically feeling for lumps all around each breast, including under the nipple and in the axilla. It is best performed in the supine position with one arm raised over the head as this spreads out the breast tissue and deeper lumps can be felt more easily. The fingers of the other hand are then moved in a small circular motion working from around the nipple area to the outer edges of the breast in concentric circles, remembering to feel in each axilla. If the woman finds anything she is concerned about, she should present to her GP for examination.

Mammography

Mammography uses X-rays to visualise the breast tissue and identify any abnormal masses or lumps. Women in the UK are invited for mammograms every 3 years between the ages of 50–70 years. Mammography gives up to 95% diagnostic accuracy on its own in women of this age.

Magnetic resonance imaging of the breasts

Breast MRI is another imaging technique that can be used to identify potentially cancerous breast lumps. However, MRI is an expensive method and, as such, is reserved for high-risk cases where there is diagnostic uncertainty.

GENETIC TESTING FOR BREAST CANCER

Genetic testing for breast cancer typically involves testing for mutations in the BRCA genes. Genetic testing is not offered to everyone, but rather to those women with a particularly high risk of developing of breast cancer. High-risk individuals are deemed (by NICE) to be those with the following present in the family history:

- One first-degree relative and one second-degree relative diagnosed before an average age of 50 years.

- Two first degree relatives diagnosed before an average age of 50 years.

- Three or more first- or second-degree relatives diagnosed at any age.

MANAGEMENT OF BREAST LUMPS

Any woman over the age of 25 years, who presents to her doctor with a new breast lump that is confirmed on examination, should be referred to a breast clinic. If there are any sinister features she should be seen within 2 weeks. In the breast clinic, both breasts and the axillae will be examined by a breast surgeon and the lump scanned by ultrasonography. A sample of tissue will be taken from the lump by fine needle aspiration and sent for histological diagnosis.

GRADE AND STAGE OF BREAST CANCER

Histological grade is a useful prognostic indicator: low-grade tumours are slow-growing and unlikely to spread; high-grade tumours are aggressive and metastasise early.

The tumour is staged using the TNM system, which stands for tumour size, lymph node spread, and presence or absence of metastasis. Using this system, breast cancer is grouped into four stages:

Stage 1 – lump with no spread.

Stage 2 – lump with axillary spread.

Stage 3 – lump with local spread (e.g. attachment to chest wall muscles or infiltration into overlying skin) with axillary spread.

Stage 4 – lump with local spread and distant metastases.

T0 means lump too small to assess. T1 is a lump less than 2 cm. T2 is a lump 2–5 cm, T3 is a lump over 5 cm in size, and T4 is spread to skin or chest wall. N0 means no spread to lymph nodes, N1 is spread to axillary nodes, N2 is spread to internal mammary nodes or multiple axillary nodes, N3 is spread to distant nodes. M0 is no metastasis, M1 is metastasis.

TREATMENT OF BREAST CANCER

Treatment options vary, but most require surgery. The procedure may be a wide local excision of the lump with axillary clearance of lymph nodes, or removal of the breast by mastectomy. Immediate breast reconstruction is usually offered. Radiotherapy and/or chemotherapy may follow.

ENDOMETRIAL CANCER

Endometrial cancer occurs almost exclusively in post-menopausal women. It often presents early as post-menopausal vaginal bleeding, or with a post-menopausal vaginal discharge. In the few women who contract the disease premenopausally, they may present with menorrhagia or intermenstrual bleeding.

INVESTIGATION OF POST-MENOPAUSAL BLEEDING

All women who present to their GP with post-menopausal bleeding should be referred to a rapid-access clinic for assessment within 2 weeks of presentation. This will involve a transvaginal ultrasound scan to assess endometrial thickness, and biopsy of the endometrium using a pipelle sampler or using out-patient hysteroscopy. Ultrasound scanning also allows visualisation of the ovaries, as a number of patients with postmenopausal bleeding will have ovarian pathology.

Risk factors for development of endometrial cancer

- Increasing age.
- Long-term exposure to unopposed oestrogens.
- Metabolic syndrome (obesity, diabetes).
- Nulliparity.
- History of breast cancer.
- Long-term use of tamoxifen.
- Hereditary non-polyposis colonic cancer.
- First-degree relative with endometrial cancer.
- The use of unopposed oestrogen as HRT

Factors protective against development of endometrial cancer

- Grand multiparity.
- Smoking.
- Oral-contraceptive use.

TREATMENT OF ENDOMETRIAL CANCER

In an otherwise well patient, treatment of choice will be total abdominal hysterectomy with bilateral salpingo-oophorectomy. For patients with extensive disease at presentation, or those unsuitable for surgery, treatment will be with radiotherapy.

OVARIAN CANCER

USEFUL WEBSITES

- Ovarian Cancer Action <www.ovarian.org.uk>.
- Ovarian Cancer Support Group <www.ovacome.org.uk>.

Ovarian cancer is a devastating illness that causes a number of vague, non-specific symptoms which make the diagnosis notoriously easy to miss. In many cases, ovarian cancer is completely asymptomatic in the early stages; therefore, ovarian cancer is often diagnosed late, when advanced disease has already taken hold. Signs and symptoms of ovarian cancer include abdominal swelling (due to ovarian size and/or ascites) and bloating which may be misdiagnosed as irritable bowel syndrome, pelvic pain or abdominal discomfort, irregular vaginal bleeding or post-menopausal bleeding, malaise, urinary symptoms due to the pressure of the ovarian mass on the bladder (such as recurrent urinary tract infection, urinary frequency or urinary retention), nausea and fatigue. An ovarian cancer can also present acutely as rupture of an ovarian cyst causing peritonitis, or torsion of the ovarian mass causing extreme pain and collapse. Some 5% of ovarian tumours are derived from the secretory cells of the ovarian stroma and are endocrinologically active, secreting hormones such as oestrogen or testosterone. Such tumours may present with virilisation. The majority of ovarian tumours are, however, derived from the surface epithelium.

Risk factors for development of ovarian cancer

Women who have experienced many years of ovulation are at higher risk of developing ovarian cancer than average; such women include the nulligravida or women who had their first child after the age of 35 years of age, and women who had an early menarche or late menopause. The Caucasian race has a higher incidence of ovarian cancer than other races. The combined oral contraceptive pill, Depo-Provera and Implanon are all contraceptive methods that suppress ovulation. As such, they are effective in decreasing the risk of developing ovarian cancer, as are pregnancies. It is unclear whether ovarian stimulants such as Clomifene have an effect on ovarian cancer development or not.

The *BRCA1* and *BRCA2* genes and the *HNPCC* gene are also linked to the risk of ovarian cancer. Overall, if a woman has one first-degree relative who has had ovarian cancer, her risk goes up about 4-fold, rising to 10-fold if she has two such relatives. Referral to a genetics centre is recommended for these cases.

Diagnosing ovarian cancer

Any woman with suspected ovarian cancer should be referred urgently to a rapid-access oncogynaecology clinic for assessment. Initial investigations will be with ultrasound scanning. Laparoscopy is required in order to confirm a diagnosis and assess abdominal spread. A CT scan will help identify the absence or presence of metastases.

Ca-125

The tumour marker Ca-125 is raised in 80% of women with ovarian cancer, but it should be remembered that it is not raised in 20%. Ca-125 is quite non-specific; it can also be raised by many conditions other than ovarian cancer, including benign ovarian cysts, endometriosis, fibroids, pelvic inflammatory disease and breast, pancreatic, colonic and gastric cancers. It is, therefore, not recommended that Ca-125 is used as a screening test for ovarian cancer by many hospital laboratories, although it is common practice among GPs and gynaecologists alike.

Ca-125 is extremely useful in monitoring response to treatment of ovarian cancer, and monitoring for relapse.

Management of ovarian cancer

Once a diagnosis of ovarian cancer is confirmed, the recommended treatment is usually a total abdominal hysterectomy, bilateral salpingo-ooporectomy and omentectomy. Those with advanced disease will need combination chemotherapy with radiotherapy as indicated. The prognosis depends on the stage of disease.

VULVAL CANCER

USEFUL WEBSITE

- RCOG Guideline on vulval cancer <www.rcog.org.uk/womens-health/
  clinical-guidance/management-vulval-cancer>.

VULVAL INTRA-EPITHELIAL NEOPLASIA

Vulval intra-epithelial neoplasia (VIN) is a precancerous skin lesion of the vulva, previously known as Bowen's disease of the vulva. VIN is not invasive cancer but may progress to become an invasive squamous cell cancer if left untreated.

Treatment is by laser ablation or surgical excision. Other treatments include 5-fluorouracil cream. Careful follow-up after treatment is essential as VIN may recur.

VULVAL CANCER

Vulval cancer is a very rare disease and, on average, a GP will only see a new case once every 10 years. Ninety percent of all vulval cancers are squamous cell carcinomas, with melanoma, Paget's disease, Bartholin's gland tumours, adenocarcinoma and basal cell carcinoma accounting for the remaining cases.

Management of vulval cancer

Any abnormal lesion on the vulva in a postmenopausal woman should be treated with suspicion and referred to a gynaecological rapid-access clinic. At the clinic, the lesion will be examined and biopsied. If positive for vulval cancer, treatment is with urgent surgical excision followed by radiotherapy. The 5-year survival rate for vulval cancer in cases with no lymph node involvement is in excess of 80%. The success of treatment falls rapidly if there has been local or distant spread, so early recognition is important.

Module 7: Fertility control

The examiners will expect you to demonstrate appropriate knowledge and attitudes in relation to sub-fertility. This includes an understanding of the epidemiology, aetiology, management and prognosis of male and female fertility problems. You will be expected to have a broad-based knowledge of investigation and management of the infertile couple in a primary care setting and appropriate knowledge of assisted reproductive techniques including and the legal and ethical implications of these procedures.

You will be expected to understand the indications, contra-indications, complications, and mode of action and efficacy of all reversible and irreversible contraceptive methods.

You will be expected to demonstrate appropriate knowledge of abortion and should be familiar with the accompanying laws related to abortion, consent, child protection and the Sexual Offences Act(s).

You will be expected to demonstrate appropriate knowledge, management skills and attitudes in relation to fertility control and termination of pregnancy. There may be conscientious objection to the acquisition of certain skills in areas of sexual and reproductive health but knowledge and appropriate attitudes as described above will be expected.

Module 7 discusses subfertility, as well as unwanted fertility (birth control). All contraceptive methods available in the UK are explained and the benefits for each method outlined. When unwanted pregnancy occurs, the option of terminating the pregnancy is available for women in the UK, and this is explained, as well as the laws that govern abortion.

There are a number of contraceptive options available to women and couples, and the choice of which method to chose and use lies predominantly with the patient. They should be advised of the different methods available and the benefits and disadvantages of each, so that they can make an informed choice. It is important that the woman feels in control of her choice so that she is happy with her method, and uses it successfully. NICE guidance advises that clinicians advise a long-term contraceptive method as this is more cost-effective.

There is a list of rules, or suitability criteria, that must be adhered to when prescribing contraceptives. These rules have been summarised in a very useful format known as the UK Medical Eligibility Criteria (UKMEC). The data in Tables 7.1–7.3 are invaluable when assessing risks and benefits of any contraceptive method and can be used as a

Table 7.1 Safe use of the combined oral contraceptive pill

Clinical Feature	UKMEC 1 No restrictions	UKMEC 2 Benefits generally outweigh risks	UKMEC 3 Requires expert clinical judgement	UKMEC 4 Contra-indicated
Age (years)	< 40	> 40		
Smoking	Non-smoker	Age < 35 years smoker	Age > 35 years smoker	Smoker with concurrent ischaemic heart disease or previous stroke
Obesity (BMI kg/m^2)	< 30	30–34	35–39	> 40
Hypertension	Normotensive	History of gestational hypertension	Controlled hypertension	Systolic BP > 160 or diastolic BP > 95 or hypertensive retinopathy
Other risk factors of thrombosis	Varicose veins	Superficial thrombophlebitis	Family history of thrombosis in first degree relative before relative reached age of 45 years	History of transient ischaemic attack or stroke, intermittent claudication, lupus anticoagulant
Breastfeeding	> 6 months post-partum	>6 weeks post-partum, mixed feeding	>6 weeks post-partum exclusive breast feeding	< 6 weeks post-partum
Ectopic pregnancy	History of ectopic pregnancy			
Migraine	Non-migrainous head-aches, mild or severe	Migraine without aura aged < 35 yrs	Migraine without aura aged > 35 years	Migraine with aura
Depression	Current or past depression			
Breast cancer	Family history of breast cancer; benign breast disease		History of breast cancer and no recurrence over past 5 years; carriers of *BRCA1* or *BRCA2* gene mutations	
Abnormal vaginal bleeding	Irregular bleeding, but not suspicious	Unexplained vaginal bleeding suspicious of serious underlying condition	Enzyme-inducing drugs such as barbiturates, carbamazepine, griseofulvin, phenytoin, rifampicin	
Medications		Antibiotic that is not enzyme inducing; HAART		
Surgery	History of pelvic surgery, or any surgery without immobilisation	Surgery without prolonged immobilisation		Surgery with prolonged immobilisation
Gynaecological conditions	Endometriosis; cervical ectroption; uterine fibroids; PID	CIN and cervical cancer		Gestational trophoblastic disease
Non-gynaecological conditions	Thyroid disease	Sickle-cell anaemia; gall-bladder disease; HIV/AIDS using HAART; uncomplicated diabetes; hyperlipidaemia	History of cholestasis; diabetes with complications	Active viral hepatitis

Adapted from UK Medical Eligibility Criteria for use of combined oral contraceptives; full guidance can be downloaded from <http://www.ffprhc.org.uk/admin/uploads/298_UKMEC_200506.pdf>.

Table 7.2 Safe use of the progestogen-only pill

Clinical Feature	UKMEC 1 No restrictions	UKMEC 2 Benefits generally outweigh risks	UKMEC 3 Requires expert clinical judgement	UKMEC 4 Contra-indicated
Age	Menarche – menopause			
Smoking	Smokers and non-smokers			
Obesity	All weights			
Hypertension	All blood pressures	Hypertensive retinopathy		
Other risk factors thrombosis	Family history or personal history of thrombosis	Current thrombosis; known thombophilic mutations; Raynaud's disease with lupus anticoagulant		
Breast-feeding	Breast-feeding at any time post-partum			
Ectopic pregnancy	History of ectopic pregnancy			
Migraine	Non-migrainous headaches	Migraine without aura	Migraine with aura	
Depression	Current or past depression			
Breast cancer	Family history of breast cancer; benign breast disease	Undiagnosed breast mass	History of breast cancer and no recurrence over past 5 years	Current breast cancer
Abnormal vaginal bleeding		Unexplained abnormal vaginal bleeding		
Medications	Antibiotics that are not enzyme inducing	HAART anti-viral drugs	Enzyme inducing drugs such as barbiturates, carbimazapine, griseofulvin, phenytoin, rifampicin	
Surgery	Major surgery without prolonged immobilisation	Major surgery with prolonged immobilisation		
Gynaecological conditions	Cervical cancer; endometrial cancer; ovarian cancer; uterine fibroids; endometriosis			
Non-gynaecological conditions	Sickle-cell disease; thyroid disease; diabetes without complications	Hyperlipidaemia; diabetes with complications; history of cholestasis	Active viral hepatitis; decompensated liver disease	

Adapted from UK Medical Eligibility Criteria for use of combined oral contraceptives; full guidance can be downloaded from <http://www.ffprhc.org.uk/admin/uploads/298_UKMEC_200506.pdf>.

Table 7.3 Safe use of the intra-uterine device

Clinical Feature	UKMEC 1 No restrictions	UKMEC 2 Benefits generally outweigh risks	UKMEC 3 Requires expert clinical judgement	UKMEC 4 Contra-indicated
Age (years)	> 20 – Menopause	Menarche – 20		
Parity	Parous, non-parous			
Smoking	Smoker or non-smoker			
Obesity	Any weight			
Hypertension	Any blood pressure; hypertensive retinopathy			
Other risk factors thrombosis	Past thrombosis; carrier of thrombophilic mutations		Current thrombosis on anti-coagulants	
Breast-feeding	Breast-feeding at any time post-partum			
Ectopic pregnancy	History of ectopic pregnancy			
Migraine	Migraine with aura			
Depression	Current or past depression			
Breast cancer	Current or past breast cancer			
Abnormal vaginal bleeding	Irregular periods	Heavy or prolonged menstrual bleeding		Unexplained vaginal bleeding suspicious of serious underlying condition
Medications	Enzyme-inducing drugs	HAART anti-retroviral drugs		
Surgery	Major surgery with or without prolonged immobilisation			
Gynaecological conditions	Cervical ectropian; CIN	Severe dysmenorrhoea; endometriosis; cervical cancer; endometrial cancer; current PID (if IUD already *in situ*)	Ovarian cancer	Gestational trophoblastic disease; uterine abnormality that distorts the uterine cavity; current PID (if IUD not yet *in situ*)
Non-gynae-cological conditions	Ischaemic heart disease; gallbladder disease; viral hepatitis; diabetes; thyroid disease	Iron-deficiency anaemia; thalassaemia; sickle-cell disease		

Adapted from UK Medical Eligibility Criteria for use of combined oral contraceptives; full guidance can be downloaded from <http://www.ffprhc.org.uk/admin/uploads/298_UKMEC_200506.pdf>.

reference, but it is important to refer regularly to the Faculty of Sexual and Reproductive Healthcare (FSHR) website for any new or up-dated guidance.

USEFUL WEBSITES

- Written information leaflets on all of the contraceptive methods available for use in the UK can be accessed on <www.patient.co.uk>.

- Full and condensed UKMEC guidelines from the Faculty of Family Planning and Reproductive Health Care can be accessed on <www.ffprhc.org.uk>.

- Full downloadable UK Medical Eligibility Criteria can be found at <http://www.ffprhc.org.uk/admin/uploads/298_UKMEC_200506.pdf>.

- Or a summary can be found at <http://www.cks.nhs.uk/contraception/management/detailed_answers/uk_medical_eligibility_criteria>

THE COMBINED ORAL CONTRACEPTIVE

Since the introduction of the combined oral contraceptive (COC) pill in 1960, the life of women has been revolutionised. Often simply referred to as 'the pill', combined oral contraceptives were welcomed by many women as an opportunity for real freedom from unwanted pregnancies. Until the introduction of combined oral contraceptives, for many women the only way of avoiding pregnancy was to abstain from sex; this is far easier said than done, and is often out of the woman's control. 'The pill' was first introduced in the USA, and its popularity there rapidly spread across the globe. Combined oral contraceptives are now taken by over 100 million women world-wide each year.

HOW THE COMBINED ORAL CONTRACEPTIVE WORKS

The COC provides serum levels of oestrogen and progestogen sufficient to inhibit release of FSH and LH from the anterior pituitary gland, and consequently prevents ovulation. As long as ovulation is suppressed, fertilisation will be impossible. As well as preventing ovulation, the progestogen acts on the endometrium to reduce its receptiveness to implantation and causes thickening of the cervical mucus decreasing its permeability to sperm. Many women find that their periods become lighter and less painful when taking the COC and it is sometimes used for this purpose alone, particularly in young girls who have not yet embarked on any sexual activity.

When the COC is discontinued, fertility can return immediately. For some women there is a delay of 2–3 months until full baseline fertility is achieved, so there is great variability in this. Many women become pregnant on just missing two or three pills, and it is important to ensure that the woman understands that taking the pill regularly is essential if she wants to prevent pregnancy.

ADVANTAGES OF TAKING THE COC

- Reduction in menstrual blood loss. The COC can be used as a treatment for menorrhagia.

- Reduction in menstrual pain. The COC can be used as a treatment for endometriosis.

- Predictable regular withdrawal bleeds, and the possibility of postponing bleeds if the timing would be inconvenient.

- Improvement in facial complexion. Any COC can be used as a treatment for acne, but the results vary between women.

- Possible protection against osteoporosis.

- A 50% reduction in the risk of ovarian cancer and ovarian cysts. This protection continues for over 15 years after COC use has ceased.

- A 50% reduction in the risk of endometrial cancer. This protection continues for over 15 years after COC use has ceased.

- Reduction in benign breast disease.

- Vastly reduced likelihood of ectopic pregnancy.

DISADVANTAGES OF TAKING THE COC

No protection against STIs with COC

The COC provides no protection against sexually transmitted infections. This is important to consider, particularly in young couples who may feel that the female partner being 'on the pill' means that they are free to have unprotected sex, and the female or male partner may be coerced into doing so using this argument. It is, therefore, important to emphasise that condoms should be used, along with taking the pill, unless the couple is in a stable exclusive relationship.

Risk of venous thrombosis with COC

The relative risk of venous thrombosis is five times higher in COC users when compared to non-COC using females. It must be remembered that the absolute risk is still very low, and considerably lower than the risk of venous thrombosis in pregnancy.

- *Healthy non-pregnant women* – 5 cases per 100,000 woman years.

- *COC users* – 15–25 per 100,000 per year depending on the type of progestogen used.

- *Pregnancy* – 60 per 100,000 per year.

All of these risks increase with increasing age, and the risk is compounded if other risk factors for thrombosis are present.

Risk of myocardial infarction and ischaemic stroke with COC

Healthy non-smokers have no increased risk of myocardial infarction with COC use. COC users with hypertension have a 3-fold increased risk of myocardial infarction compared with COC users without hypertension. COC users who are heavy smokers (more than 15 cigarettes per day) have a 10-fold increased risk of myocardial infarction compared to smokers who do not use the COC.

There is a very small increase in the risk of ischaemic stroke with COC use.

Risk of cervical cancer with COC

The risk of developing cervical cancer is very slightly increased after at least 5 years of COC usage. It is not clear whether this is due to the pill itself, or the fact that COC users are more likely to be having unprotected sex and are thus more exposed to the HPV virus. Women should be encourage to join in the national cervical screening programme.

Risk of breast cancer with COC

One in nine women will develop breast cancer at some time in their lives. Any extra risk of breast cancer caused by the COC is likely to be small, will vary with age and be gone 10 years after stopping the combined pill.

ABSOLUTE CONTRA-INDICATIONS TO THE COC PILL

- Breast feeding at less than 6 weeks' post-partum. This is because the COC at this early stage reduces breast-milk volume. There is little evidence that this effect continues after 6 post-partum weeks, but most clinicians do not prescribe the COC pill until breast-feeding has ceased, or the baby is 6 months of age.

- Obesity with a body mass index over 40 kg/m^2.

- Age ≥ 35 years and smoking ≥ 15 cigarettes daily.

- Multiple risks for arterial cardiovascular disease

- A history of venous thrombo-embolism, and/or a known clotting disorder.

- Major surgery with prolonged immobilisation.

- A history of ischaemic heart disease, ischaemic stroke or peripheral vascular disease.

- A history of complicated congenital or valvular heart disease, e.g. heart disease with pulmonary hypertension, atrial fibrillation, endocarditis etc. (in uncomplicated heart disease, it can be prescribed).

- Systolic blood pressure ≥ 160 bpm, or diastolic blood pressure ≥ 95 (in controlled hypertensives it can be prescribed, but other contraceptive methods are very preferable – UKMEC 3).

- A history of migraine with aura. Aura includes homonymous hemi-anopia, visual fortification spectra or scotoma, unilateral weakness, paraesthesia or numbness, and speech disorder. (Note that flashing lights do not count as aura).

- Current breast cancer.

- Active viral hepatitis, acute porphyria, severe decompensating liver failure, or liver cancer.

- Gestational trophoblastic disease.

- Diabetes with complications, or of more than 20 years' duration.

DIFFERENT PREPARATIONS OF THE COC PILL

There are a number of different preparations on the market. Table 7.4 shows the combined oral contraceptive pills available in the UK.

HOW TO TAKE THE COC PILL

Ideally, the first COC pill should be taken on the first day of the woman's menstrual period. A pill is then taken every day for 21 days, followed by a 7-day, pill-free interval (or 7 days of placebo tablets for the everyday preparations). During the pill-free interval, most women will experience a withdrawal bleed as long as they are not pregnant. After 7 pill-free days, a new packet of the pill should be started regardless of whether the withdrawal bleed has completed or not. It is important to emphasise this to the user, as it is thought that the majority of missed pills occur due to late starting of the new packet, and some women may hold the false belief that conception is impossible while menstruating. It should be pointed out that every strip should be started on the same day of the week, i.e. a 'Wednesday girl' should always start her new packet on a Wednesday.

The COC can be started mid-cycle if there has not been any sex since the last period, and condoms are used until she has taken 7 consecutive pills.

CHOICE OF COC PILL

As shown in Table 7.4, COCs vary in the quantity of ethinyloestradiol and in the type and quantity of progestogen. All the pills are equally effective in avoiding pregnancy; the typical-use pregnancy rate among COC users varies depending on the population being studied, ranging from 2–8% per year. The perfect-use pregnancy rate of COCs is 0.3% per year.

For first-time users, a levonorgestrel or norethisterone pill is first choice; this is because these formulations are 'second-generation' progestogens which carry the lowest risk of venous thrombosis. The COC usually prescribed first-line to women in the UK is Microgynon, but Ovysmen is half the price and most women settle nicely to its use.

Table 7.4 The combined oral contraceptive pills available in the UK

Name	Oestrogen mcg	Progesterone mcg
Low oestrogen pills		
Femodette	Ethinyloestradiol 20	Gestodene 75
Loestrin 20	Ethinyloestradiol 20	Noreithisterone 1000
Mercilon	Ethinyloestradiol 20	Desogestrel 150
Sunya 20/75	Ethinyloestradiol 20	Gestodene 75
Medium oestrogen pills		
Brevinor	Ethinyloestradiol 35	Noreithisterone 500
Cilest	Ethinyloestradiol 35	Norgestimate 250
Dianette	Ethinyloestradiol 35	Cyproterone acetate 2000
Femodene, Femodene ED	Ethinyloestradiol 30	Gestodene 75
Katya 30/75	Ethinyloestradiol 30	Gestodene 75
Loestrin 30	Ethinyloestradiol 30	Noreithisterone 1500
Marvelon	Ethinyloestradiol 30	Desogestrel 150
Microgynon 30,	Ethinyloestradiol 30	Levonorgestrel 150
Microgynon 30 ED,	Ethinyloestradiol 30	Levonorgestrel 150
Ovranette	Ethinyloestradiol 30	Levonorgestrel 150
Minulet	Ethinyloestradiol 30	Gestodene 75
Norimin	Ethinyloestradiol 35	Noreithisterone 1000
Ovysmen	Ethinyloestradiol 35	Noreithisterone 500
Yasmin	Ethinyloestradiol 30	Drospirenone 30
High oestrogen pills		
Norinyl-1	Mestranol 50	Noreithisterone 1000
Cyclical pills		
Binovum	Ethinyloestradiol 35	Norethisterone 500, 1000
Logynon	Ethinyloestradiol 30, 40, 30	Levonorgestrel 50, 75, 125
Logynon ED	Ethinyloestradiol 30, 40, 30	Levonorgestrel 50, 75, 125
Synphase	Ethinyloestradiol 35	Norethisterone 500, 1000, 500
Triadene	Ethinyloestradiol 30, 40, 30	Gestodene 50, 70, 100
Tri-Minulet	Ethinyloestradiol 30, 40, 30	Gestodene 50, 70, 100
TriNovum	Ethinyloestradiol 35	Noreithisterone 500, 1000, 500

Microgynon also comes in an everyday preparation with placebo tablets to assist those who become confused by having a 'week break'.

A new preparation, Qlaira, has a 'natural' oestrogen (oestradiol valerate) as opposed to the synthetic oestrogens used in other preparations. The rules for its use are somewhat different, but contra-indications are the same as for other combined pills. Qlaira is rather expensive. Its role has yet to be established.

CHOICE OF PILL FOR WOMEN WITH ACNE OR HIRSUTISM

For women with acne or hirsutism, any combined oral contraceptive may help. It may be necessary to try different types to find the best one for the individual woman. Drosperinone-containing contraceptives, such as Yasmin or Yaz, are frequently used but are very expensive.

Co-cyprindiol (e.g. Dianette or Clairette) is not recommended solely for contraceptive use. It is, however, licensed for treatment of severe acne refractory to oral antibiotics and for moderately severe hirsutism. Formation of venous thrombosis is four times more likely on Co-cyprindiol when compared to Microgynon, it should be withdrawn 3–4 months after the symptoms have settled.

COC PILL RULES

As long as the pill rules are followed correctly, the woman will be protected from pregnancy, even during the pill-free week.

Missed pills

A woman has 24 hours in which to remember to take her pill each day. If she is more than 24 hours late taking her pill, it will be classed as a 'missed pill'.

If one or more pills are missed within the first seven of the packet, precautions (condoms, diaphragm or abstinence) need to be taken until seven consecutive pills have been taken. If unprotected sex has occurred, emergency contraception should be offered.

If one or two pills are missed during the second week, no extra precautions are required and the woman should be advised to restart taking the pill. If one or two pills are missed during the third week, no extra precautions are required, but the next packet should be started without taking a pill-free week. For the minority of patients who take the low-dose oestrogen pills Loestrin, Mercilon or Femodette, there is only room to miss one pill in the first or third week without risking pregnancy.

Antibiotics

Some broad-spectrum antibiotics (such as amoxicillin and doxycycline) may reduce the efficacy of combined oral contraceptives by impairing the bacterial flora responsible for recycling of ethinyloestradiol from the large bowel. Advice is that additional contraceptive precautions are needed whilst taking a short course of a broad-spectrum antibiotic and for 7 days after the antibiotic course is complete. If these 7 days run beyond the end of a packet, the next packet should be started without a break.

Gastrointestinal illness

Any gastrointestinal illness that causes diarrhoea or vomiting will disrupt absorbance of the COC pill through the gut, and render it less effective depending on the severity and duration of the illness. The COC pill is, therefore, not appropriate for those who suffer from chronic diarrhoeal illnesses such as Crohn's disease or ulcerative colitis, or those with a shortened gut. For patients on the COC who experience a brief infectious gastroenteritis, advice is that the woman should continue to take the COC as normal, but that extra contraceptive precautions should be taken for the duration of the illness and subsequent 7 days.

Enzyme-inducing drugs

Hepatic enzyme-inducing drugs (such as some anti-epileptic medications, rifamycins, and some anti-retrovirals) reduce the efficacy of COCs by breaking them down more quickly. This effect lasts for 28 days after the last dose is taken. As a result, oral contraceptives are not generally recommended for women taking such medications. The complementary medicine St John's Wort is also an enzyme inducer, it is sold without prescription and women on combined or progestogen-only pills, or progestogen implants, need to be warned against its use.

AVOIDING WITHDRAWAL BLEEDS

Women who wish to avoid a withdrawal bleed may take two or three packets of the pill consecutively, missing the week breaks in between, and thus postponing the withdrawal bleed. Some women choose to take three packets in a row routinely, thus having only four periods a year. This is known as tricycling and is particularly helpful for endometriosis sufferers, women with menstrual migraines or psychotic symptoms precipitated by menstruation.

Tricycling is not known to be harmful in any way; thus, this method may be used by women who simply dislike the cost and inconvenience of regular monthly menstruation.

THE CONTRACEPTIVE PATCH

> **USEFUL WEBSITE**
>
> - <www.orthoevra.com>.

The contraceptive patch, Evra, is relatively new to the market. It is a 20 cm × 20 cm patch that is put on the skin to allow transdermal absorption of hormones. It releases 20 mcg of ethinyloestradiol and 150 mcg of norelgestromin every 24 hours.

INSTRUCTIONS ON USAGE OF THE CONTRACEPTIVE PATCH

One patch is applied on the skin on the first day of menstruation. The patch is removed and replaced on the same day each week for the next 2 weeks, followed by a patch-free week. During the patch-free week, most women experience a withdrawal bleed if not pregnant. If the woman forgets to change the patch on day 7, evidence suggests that she will be protected for a further 2 days.

The patch can be placed on any flat surface of the body apart from the breasts, face, soles or palms. It is very sticky and is designed to stay on in the bath, shower, swimming pool, and during sweaty exercise. It is recommended that each patch should be placed on a different area of skin each week in order to avoid contact sensitivity. The contraceptive patch can lighten the skin colour of dark-skinned women under the patch if the patch is continuously placed on the same spot.

Patch prescribing

It is recommended that use of the contraceptive patch is restricted to those women who are likely to comply poorly with a COC pill; this is mainly because the patch is more expensive than the pill. Compliance with the patch has been shown to be better than taking a daily pill.

The contraceptive patch carries the same risks and benefits of the COC pill and the same contra-indications apply. There is thought to be a slightly higher risk of venous thrombosis on the patch than the pill as the woman receives a higher dose of oestrogen.

PATCH RULES

If the patch comes off and it has been off for less than 48 hours, a new patch should be applied and no further precautions are required. The next patch should be changed on the normal patch change day to avoid confusion.

If the patch comes off and it has been off for over 48 hours, a new patch cycle should be started by applying a fresh patch as soon as possible. This would then become the new patch change day, week one. Extra contraceptive precautions should be taken for 7 days. Emergency contraception should be offered if appropriate. Extra precautions should be used during a course of antibiotics and subsequent 7 days. No extra precautions are required if the woman experiences a diarrhoeal or vomiting illness.

Breakthrough bleeding is quite common when first starting on the patch. This usually settles down within the first 3 months but, as with any woman presenting with irregular bleeding, chlamydial infection should be excluded and a cervical smear test should be taken if one is due.

NUVA RING

USEFUL WEBSITE

- Nuva ring information <www.nuvaring.com>.

The Nuva ring is a new contraceptive method that is seldom used, but GPs should be aware of its existence. It is a vaginal ring that releases a combined hormonal preparation of oestrogen and progestogen. The Nuva ring is a flexible, plastic ring that is inserted into the vagina for 3 weeks then removed for a week to allow a withdrawal bleed.

The Nuva ring carries the same risks and benefits as the COC pill.

PROGESTOGEN-ONLY METHODS

THE PROGESTOGEN-ONLY PILL

There are five different progesterone-only pills available in the UK – Cerazette, Femulen, Micronor, Norgeston, and Noriday (Table 7.5).

Advantages of the progestogen-only pill

The progesterone-only pill (POP) is often the choice taken by women who would like to take a daily pill in order to control their fertility, but who are unsuitable for the combined oral contraceptive pill due to contra-indications. The POP is a very safe choice and suitable for almost all women, regardless of age, weight, blood pressure or concurrent illness. There are no absolute contra-indications apart from current breast cancer. It is safe to take while breast-feeding.

Table 7.5 The four progesterone-only pills available in the UK

Name	Progesterone mcg
Cerazette	Desogestrel 75
Micronor	Noreithisterone 350
Norgeston	Levonorgestrel 30
Noriday	Noreithisterone 350
Femulen	Etynodiol diacetate 500

Disadvantages of the progestogen-only pill

The main complaint of women taking the POP is that their periods can become irregular or cease completely. Troublesome bleeding may be improved by trying a different POP, or by taking two pills daily. Another disadvantage of the POP is that it has a higher failure rate in young women. It is also inactivated by enzyme-inducing drugs, see the note under combined oral contraceptives.

HOW THE PROGESTOGEN-ONLY PILL WORKS

There are three main actions by which POP prevents pregnancy:

- The POP causes thickening of the cervical mucus; this acts as a mechanical barrier, preventing the entry of sperm into the uterus.
- Ovulation is inhibited in 60% of standard POP users, and 97% of Cerazette users.
- There is an atrophy of the endometrium, rendering it hostile to implantation.

PROGESTOGEN-ONLY PILL RULES

As with the COC, it is ideal if the woman starts the POP on the first day of her menstrual period. If started as such, she will have instant contraceptive protection. The POP can be started mid-cycle if there has been no sex since the previous menstrual period, and she is aware that contraceptive protection will not start until three consecutive pills have been taken successfully.

The POP is taken everyday without any break, whether the woman is bleeding or not. With Micronor, Noriday, Femulen and Norgeston, there is only a 3-hour interval in which the woman must remember to take her pill. If she is more than 3 hours late, this is classed as a missed pill. In such circumstances, she should be advised to take the missed pill as soon as she remembers, and to use additional contraceptive precautions for the following 2 days. For diarrhoeal or vomiting illnesses, the woman should be advised to continue taking the POP as normal, but to use extra contraceptive precautions for the duration of the illness and subsequent 2 days.

GOOD PRACTICE POINT 7.1

- Remember that it is normal to have no periods or irregular periods on the progestogen-only pill. As long as the woman is sure that there have been no missed pills, there is no need to do a pregnancy test.

CERAZETTE

Cerazette is the only POP pill that reliably suppresses ovulation. As such, users enjoy a 12-hour missed-pill window, making Cerazette a popular choice for young, highly fertile women, women who work shifts or simply those with more hectic or disorganised lives.

INJECTABLE PROGESTOGENS

There are currently two injectable progestogens available for use as contraceptives – Depo-provera and Noristerat. Depo-provera is given at 12-week intervals, and Noristerat at 8-week intervals. Apart from that, they are comparable. Injectable progestogens are useful for women who cannot remember to take a pill, and who want a reliable method of contraception. As with the POP, there are no absolute contra-indications apart from current breast cancer, and injectable progestogens are suitable for most women.

Advantages of injectable progestogens

- Injectable progestogens are extremely effective. They have a failure rate of less than 1 in 1000.

- They are extremely safe.

- There is a degree of leeway as to when injections can be given, which makes injectable progestogens very convenient for the user. Depo-provera can be given any time between 10–12 weeks, 5 days after the last injection (or 14 weeks unlicensed, but known to be safe).

- Injectable progestogens are unaffected by liver enzyme-inducing drugs, and injection intervals need not be reduced.

- Injectable progestogens are unaffected by antibiotics or gastrointestinal illness.

Disadvantages of injectable progestogens

- Periods will become irregular, or may cease altogether. Many women enjoy this, but others do not.

- There may be up to one year of subfertility following use of injectable progestogen. There is great variability between women, but some women may remain amenorrhoeic for many months following use. This does not need investigation, but is an important point for women in their 30s who are planning a pregnancy, as natural fertility decreases in the late 30s.

- For women with risk factors for osteoporosis, long-term use of injectable progestogen can lead to decreased bone density. Risk factors to consider include heavy smoking, steroid use, long-term heparin use and a family history of osteoporosis. Injectable progestogens should be used with caution in young girls who are still growing (up to 18 years of age). The Committee on Safety of Medicines advice is that no laboratory tests, hormone levels, or bone-density measurements are required for the use of injectable progestogens unless risk factors for osteoporosis are present.

- Some women experience weight gain with injectable progestogens.

- Injectable progestogens provide no protection against sexually transmitted infections.

THE CONTRACEPTIVE IMPLANT

Implanon is the implantable contraceptive device available in the UK. Implanon is a flexible, subdermal rod that is highly effective in preventing pregnancy. It is easily inserted into the medial upper arm by a trained individual, and can remain in place for up to 3 years. The Implanon rod releases the progestogen, etonogestrel, steadily over the 3-year period. After 3 years, the rod is removed, and can be immediately replaced by a new one.

USEFUL WEBSITES

- Patient information <www.patient.co.uk/health/Implanon-The-Contraceptive-Implant.htm>.

- Information from Organon
  <http://www.organon.co.uk/products/gynaecology/contraception/implanon.asp>.

- Insertion and removal instruction <www.implanonlocalization.com/>.

MECHANISM OF ACTION OF THE CONTRACEPTIVE IMPLANT

Implanon works by suppressing ovulation. There is also thickening of the cervical mucus, and suppression of endometrial growth, but suppression of ovulation is the main mechanism of action. It has a failure rate of less than one in 1000.

CONTRA-INDICATIONS TO THE CONTRACEPTIVE IMPLANT

As with the POP and injectable progestogens, the contraceptive implant has no absolute contra-indications apart from current breast cancer, and is a safe choice for almost all women. However, it is inactivated by enzyme-inducing drugs, see the note under combined oral contraceptives.

SIDE-EFFECTS OF THE CONTRACEPTIVE IMPLANT

The main problem associated with Implanon is irregular bleeding. This can be quite problematic for some women, and may result in a request for early removal. Acne and/or local effects on the arm may also occur.

GOOD PRACTICE POINT 7.2

- If a woman has had an implant inserted, feel it and make sure it is still there. Routine follow-up after insertion is not recommended by NICE or the Faculty of Sexual and Reproductive Healthcare (FSRH) guidelines, but it may be wise in individual cases, especially if there is any indication for a follow-up pregnancy test. If the implant cannot be felt, assume it is not present; give emergency contraception, if indicated, and advise use of another contraceptive method until presence of the implant is confirmed by ultrasound scan.

NORPLANT

Norplant is a six-rod alternative to Implanon that is available in some developing countries, particularly in Africa. It is not available in the UK, but is sometimes seen in women who have had it fitted abroad. Norplant is safe and effective to use; it can be left in place for 5 years post-insertion. Removal of Norplant requires a specialist. Jadelle and Norplant 2 are two-rod levonorgestrel implants, but again they are not licensed for use in the UK.

INTRA-UTERINE DEVICES

The intra-uterine device (also known as the IUD or simply 'the coil') is a safe, effective method of contraception, used widely world-wide (Fig. 7.1).

There are a number of copper-containing, intra-uterine devices available in the UK. The TT380 Slimline and TCu380A Quickload can be used for up to 10 years; all other copper coils can be used for 5 years. For women who have a copper IUD fitted when they are aged over 40 years, it does not need to be changed but may be left until after the menopause (1 year after if it occurs over age 50 years, 2 years after if menopause is reached before the age of 50 years).

The IUD suits the vast majority of women and should be offered as a first-line contraceptive choice, including women who have never been pregnant.

Doctors and nurses must be specifically trained in order to fit IUDs and hold a relevant certificate of competence.

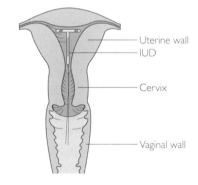

Figure 7.1 An intra-uterine device *in situ*.

MECHANISM OF ACTION OF THE IUD

The copper of the IUD has a toxic effect on sperm, effectively rendering them useless. The copper also has a toxic effect upon the ovum. The copper of the IUD also causes mild inflammation of the endometrium, making it a hostile environment, unsuitable for implantation.

The IUD, even when used as a post-coital method, does not act by causing abortion. Objections on the grounds of destroying a fertilised ovum are theological, rather than medical, but should be respected.

GOOD PRACTICE POINT 7.3

- Offer the intra-uterine device to women who ask for emergency contraception, it is more effective than Levonelle. It can be used to cover all episodes of unprotected sex up to day 19 of a 28-day menstrual cycle (see Emergency contraception p159).

ADVANTAGES OF THE IUD

- Hormone free.
- Once inserted does not rely on the user to remember anything.
- Cheap.
- Fertility returns immediately on removal of the device.
- The IUD can be used as an emergency post-coital contraceptive method, as well as for long-term contraception.

DISADVANTAGES OF THE IUD

- Periods become heavier, and may become more painful.
- The IUD provides no protection against sexually transmitted infections; in the first 21 days after insertion, there is a higher risk of developing pelvic inflammatory disease (PID). After the first 21 days, the risk of pelvic inflammatory disease is the same as a woman without a coil. If PID does occur with a coil *in situ*, the woman should be treated with appropriate antibiotics. The coil should only be removed if symptoms fail to improve following at least 72 hours of treatment.
- There is a low (1 in 500) risk of perforation of the uterus on insertion of the device.
- There is a failure rate of 1–2% if used over 5 years. If pregnancy does occur with the IUD and the threads can be seen, the IUD should be removed as this will reduce the risk of late miscarriage. If threads are not seen, the woman should have an ultrasound scan. If the IUD and the fetus are both within the uterine cavity, the IUD will be left in place and the woman will be given the choice of continuing with the pregnancy or proceeding to termination. There will be a slightly higher risk of second trimester miscarriage if the woman decides to carry a pregnancy with an IUD *in situ*, but usually the outcome is good, and the IUD will be sought at delivery.
- Expulsion, if it does occur, most often happens within the first couple of months of insertion. For this reason, women are taught how to check the threads of their device and to attend for an IUD check 3–6 weeks after fitting.
- Should an IUD fail, one in five of pregnancies will be ectopic. It is important to remember that the overall risk of ectopic pregnancy is much lower in IUD users than in women who do not use contraception; previous ectopic pregnancy is not a contra-indication to IUD use.

- Some women do not like the idea of something in their womb and are scared of the fitting procedure. Women can be assured that the IUD can be uncomfortable to insert, but is usually not painful, and the procedure only takes about 10 minutes.

ABSOLUTE CONTRA-INDICATIONS TO IUD INSERTION

- Confirmed or possible pregnancy.

- Current pelvic inflammatory disease including pelvic tuberculosis, or any signs/symptoms of a sexually transmitted infection.

- Uterine fibroids that distort the uterine cavity.

- Known uterine anomaly that distorts the uterine cavity.

- Cervical or endometrial cancer.

THE INTRA-UTERINE SYSTEM

USEFUL WEBSITES

- Mirena <www.mirena-us.com>.

- *NICE Guidance Heavy Menstrual Bleeding* <www.nice.org.uk/CG044>.

The intrauterine system (IUS) is also known as the Mirena coil. It has become extremely fashionable in recent years, and has revolutionised the treatment of menorrhagia. The IUS is very similar in appearance to the IUD but does not contain any copper; rather, on its stem, it carries the progestogen levonorgestrel which it secretes slowly over 5 years.

MECHANISM OF ACTION OF THE IUS

It is not known exactly why the Mirena is so highly effective in preventing pregnancy, displaying a failure rate lower than that of the IUD or female sterilisation, particularly as over 75% of users continue to ovulate. It is clear that the Mirena coil causes marked atrophy of the endometrium making it unsuitable for implantation. If that was the main mechanism of action, one would still expect a similar ectopic pregnancy rate to that of IUD users, which is not the case. The ectopic pregnancy rate with the Mirena coil is negligible. It is likely that the main mechanism of action is that of levonorgestrel on the endometrium causing atrophy, and on the cervix causing thickening of the cervical mucus which prevents the passage of sperm into the uterine cavity. It is also likely that transport of sperm into the fallopian tubes is also prevented.

THE IUS AS A TREATMENT FOR MENORRHAGIA

The Mirena coil results in a great reduction in the volume of blood lost during menstruation and is recommended by NICE as the first-line treatment for menorrhagia. Irregular bleeding commonly occurs during the first 3–6 months of use but, by 12 months of use, menstrual bleeding has been reduced by up to 90%, and one in five women experience amenorrhoea.

SIDE-EFFECTS OF IUS USE

Some women experience mastalgia, headaches, acne and nausea with the Mirena coil, but research has shown that these symptoms are equally as common in IUD users. These symptoms usually settle after 3 months of use.

BARRIER METHODS

CONDOMS

Condoms, in some form or another, have been used successfully to prevent pregnancy for thousands of years, and are still very popular today. Condoms are the only contraceptive method that has the massive advantage of providing protection against sexually transmitted infections. Because of this, couples are encouraged to use condoms regularly in addition to a long-term reliable contraceptive method. Condoms come in all shapes, sizes, colours and flavours. There are no contra-indications. There are latex-free condoms available for those allergic to latex. Water-based lubricant can be used with condoms if required, but oil-based lubricants should be avoided as they can damage the condom.

Condoms come in male and female versions (Fig. 7.2). The male condom is far more popular. The failure rate of condoms varies greatly with the user group. If used properly and consistently, male condoms have a failure rate of less than 2%.

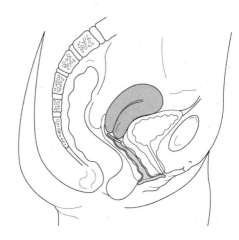

Figure 7.2 The female condom *in situ*.

GOOD PRACTICE POINT 7.4

- When giving out free condoms, always check that the patient knows how to use them properly. Poor or late application of the condom, or use of oil-based lubricants can result in splitting or failure of the condom.

Advantages of condoms

- Condoms are the most easily accessible contraceptive method, being available for purchase from chemists, supermarkets, petrol stations, and self-service machines in public toilets. Condoms are provided free by most GP surgeries and all family planning clinics. Condoms are also provided free in most university halls of residence and student unions.
- Condoms provide some protection against all sexually transmitted infections.
- Condoms reduce the risk of developing cervical neoplasia.
- Condoms are hormone free.
- Condoms are liked by some as there is 'less mess' after sex, as semen can all be discarded neatly inside the used condom.
- Condoms are helpful for men who complain of premature ejaculation as their use can lengthen time taken to ejaculation by decreasing friction.
- Condom use helps to reduce the smell from alkaline semen.

Disadvantages of condoms

- Some couples, particularly men, feel that condoms reduce the sensation and pleasure of sex.
- Some couples feel that putting the condom on interrupts sex.
- Condoms require discipline and are strongly reliant on the male partner.

DIAPHRAGMS AND CAPS

Diaphragms (Fig. 7.3) and the cervical cap Femcap (Fig. 7.4) are available in the UK, but are not used often. They require fitting and the woman needs to be trained in how to use the method. However, once trained, there are many women who enjoy using the diaphragm or cap.

USE OF SPERMICIDE WITH THE DIAPHRAGM OR CAP

The diaphragm and Femcap should always be used with a spermicidal cream, which is applied to the device prior to insertion. They should be left in place for a minimum of 6 hours after sex. If sex is repeated within 6 hours, more spermicide should be used.

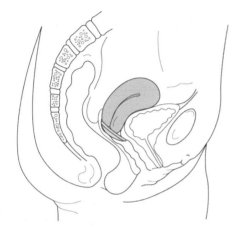

Figure 7.3 The diaphragm *in situ*.   **Figure 7.4** Femcap *in situ*.

ADVANTAGES OF THE DIAPHRAGM AND CAP

- They are hormone free.
- Unlike the male condom, neither the diaphragm nor cap relies on the male partner.
- Use of the diaphragm and cap reduces the risk of developing cervical neoplasia.

DISADVANTAGES OF THE DIAPHRAGM AND CAP

- There is a higher failure rate (4–8% for diaphragms) when compared to other contraceptive methods.
- Some women find the use of spermicide messy.
- The woman (or her partner) must be comfortable examining herself internally, and must be competent in fitting the device properly.
- There is a small, increased risk of developing urinary tract infections.
- The diaphragm cannot be used if there is any uterovaginal prolapse, poor perineal tone, neither can be used if there is a past history of toxic shock syndrome.
- Vaginal soreness can occur if the wrong size is used. A new size may be required if the woman loses or gains weight.

EMERGENCY (POST-COITAL) CONTRACEPTION

LEVONELLE

Levonorgestrel can be taken at a dose of 1500 mcg as a post-coital method of contraception. It comes as a tablet called Levonelle, and is referred to by some users as 'the morning after pill'. The effectiveness of Levonelle is greatest when taken immediately after coitus, and effectiveness declines with increasing time lapsed since coitus. Levonelle is not as effective as other contraceptive methods and, as such, should not be relied on for regular use. However, it is a good choice in the emergency situation.

When Levonelle can be used

It may be supplied if no contraceptive method was used, or if a method may have failed (forgotten pills, expelled IUDs, broken condoms, etc.).

Levonelle is licensed for use up to 72 hours post-coitus (Table 7.6) and there is some evidence that it still has an effect up to 120 hours post-coitus. A repeat dose of Levonelle should be given for each episode of unprotected sex, which may be more than once during one menstrual cycle. There is no time within the menstrual cycle when it can be certain that unprotected sex will not result in pregnancy; as such, emergency contraception should always be offered.

Table 7.6 Effectiveness of Levonelle as a function of time since coitus

Time lapsed since coitus	Expected pregnancies prevented
24 hours	95%
48 hours	85%
72 hours	58%

There are no contra-indications to use of Levonelle, and it is a safe choice for all women. Contrary to common belief, Levonelle is safe for those women with a history of ectopic pregnancy and recent evidence shows no increased risk of ectopic pregnancy following Levonelle.

Availability of Levonelle

Levonelle is available to purchase over-the-counter but must be supplied by a pharmacist. It is provided free from family planning clinics, NHS walk-in centres, hospital accident and emergency departments, and can be prescribed by GPs (or any other medical doctor) for free collection. In many areas, schemes have been set up to enable pharmacists to supply free Levonelle to selected groups of women, for example, teenagers.

Use of Levonelle by women on liver enzyme-inducing drugs

Women on liver enzyme-inducing drugs should be advised that fitting of an IUD is preferable (as long as there are no contra-indications); if the IUD is declined and Levonelle used, women should be given a double dose (i.e. 3 mg of Levonorgestrel).

Ellaone

Ellaone (ulipristal acetate) is a new, oral, post-coital contraceptive that is said to have a more sustained action over 5 days than Levonelle. Its place has yet to be established.

THE IUD AS AN EMERGENCY METHOD

The copper IUD can be inserted as an effective and safe method of post-coital contraception as it has a toxic effect on the sperm and ovum, thus preventing fertilisation. The IUD can be inserted up to 5 days' post-coitus, at any time in the menstrual cycle if there has been only one episode of unprotected sex. If there has been more than one episode of unprotected sex, a copper IUD can be fitted up to 5 days after the expected ovulation day (ovulation day would be expected on day 14 of a 28-day menstrual cycle, so IUD fitting could take place as late as day 19). The IUD must not be inserted if more than 5 days have passed since coitus and it is 5 days after the expected ovulation day as the IUD is not an abortifactant and cannot be inserted if pregnancy is a possibility.

When the IUD is used as an emergency method in this way, it is up to 99% effective. There is no increased risk of ectopic pregnancy following use of the IUD. The IUD can be removed at the next period, or kept in place for long-term usage.

NATURAL FERTILITY METHODS

Fertility awareness methods are popular among women who have a conscientious or religious objection to formal contraception, yet want to avoid pregnancy. By learning when the most fertile times of the menstrual cycle are, and avoiding sex during these periods, many couples are successfully able to avoid pregnancy. When followed correctly, fertility awareness methods can be up to 98% effective.

OVULATION PREDICTION

Although a basic measure, some women with a regular menstrual cycle simply estimate the day of ovulation, and avoid unprotected sex for 5 days prior and 5 days after the expected ovulation day. The great advantage of this is that it is free and easy to do. It is far more effective than using no contraceptive precautions, but is only really suitable for couples who would not mind a pregnancy (the failure rate is higher than other methods) or have no other option available to them.

WITHDRAWAL METHOD

The withdrawal method is an age-old technique (it is even described in the Old Testament of the Bible) and its use is extremely common, far more than many doctors realise. The withdrawal method is simply the male partner ensuring that ejaculation occurs outside the woman's vagina. This method is far more effective at preventing pregnancy than use of no precautions at all, and its use should not be under-estimated. However, if a couple really does want to avoid pregnancy, a more reliable method should be chosen as the pre-ejaculate can contain up to a million sperm, which can be enough to achieve fertilisation. In addition, some men are not as good at controlling ejaculation as they would like to think and accidents can occur.

LACTATIONAL AMENORRHOEA

If a woman is fully or nearly fully breast-feeding, amenorrhoeic, and within 6 months of delivery, she can be re-assured that pregnancy is highly unlikely, as breast feeding in this way is over 98% effective in preventing pregnancy.

PERSONA

Persona is a small monitor, available for purchase from many high-street stores, which a woman can use to identify her fertile days. It involves collection of urine each morning and testing the urine with a testing strip which is inserted into the Persona monitor. A red light will show on fertile days (i.e. unprotected sex may result in pregnancy, should proceed with caution using condoms, or abstain) and a green light will show on infertile days (free to enjoy unprotected sex without the risk of pregnancy).

Persona is 94% effective when used according to instructions.

Persona restrictions

A drawback of Persona is that it really only works well for women who have regular menstrual cycles of at least 23 days and not more than 35 days; it is not suitable for women with infrequent periods, breast-feeding women, or perimenopausal women. Another disadvantage is that the monitor is expensive and is not available free on the NHS. The test-strips are also expensive and run out quite quickly.

Persona is highly reliant on the user, the woman having to check her urine regularly and meticulously. This is not convenient for many, especially for those with a more hectic life-style. Should unprotected sex occur on a 'red-light day', unwanted pregnancy will be a likely result. Should the user notice a pattern in her menstrual cycles, it is possible for her to be falsely reassured and stop monitoring the urine. In such circumstances, the occasional fluctuations which occur in all menstrual cycles could go unnoticed and result in an unwanted pregnancy.

FERTILITY AWARENESS METHODS

Fertility awareness methods combine three fertility indicators in order to identify the fertile period.

These indicators are:

- *Basal body temperature* – body temperature rises by at least 0.2°C after ovulation.

- *Cervical secretion consistency* – secretions are described as being dry prior to ovulation, clear watery and slippery around ovulation time, then thick and sticky post-ovulation.

- *Length of the menstrual cycle* – the calculation for cycle length is based on the previous 6–12 menstrual cycles. The shortest cycle minus twenty gives the first fertile day. The longest cycle minus ten gives the last fertile day.

Combining these three indicators and plotting them on a graph, clearly identifies the fertile period of each menstrual cycle; if abstinence or barrier contraception is used during the fertile days, this method is over 98% effective.

FEMALE STERILISATION

Sterilisation is a permanent method of contraception and should be thought of as irreversible. It is only suitable for women who are absolutely sure that they do not want to have any more children. Sterilisation is available to women who do not have any children, and to women under the age of 30 years but, in such cases, the gynaecologist will need to be convinced that the woman is clear on her decision, and that alternative methods have been considered and tried. Regret is highest in women who have the procedure done post-partum or immediately following termination of pregnancy.

Female sterilisation can be performed under regional or general anaesthetic. It is a quick and safe procedure that involves placement of a plastic clip onto each fallopian tube with the aid of a laparoscope. Female sterilisation is effective after the next menstrual period and is 98% successful. Should a pregnancy occur in a sterilised woman, 10% of such pregnancies will be ectopic. However, uncomplicated female sterilisation has no long-term effects on menstruation, mood, sexual performance or libido, and may give women a sense of freedom any take away the worry of 'contraception'.

VASECTOMY

Vasectomy should always be mentioned to women and couples who ask for female sterilisation. Vasectomy is safer, more effective, quicker and easier to perform than female sterilisation and, as such, is always preferred over female sterilisation as a contraceptive choice for couples. As with female sterilisation, vasectomy should

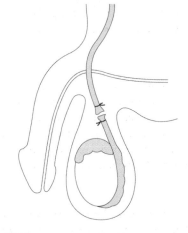

Figure 7.5 Vasectomy.

be thought of as a permanent contraceptive method that is irreversible. The male partner must be sure that he does not want to father any more children.

Vasectomy involves ligation of the vas deferens, which can also be done using a 'non-scalpel' technique under local anaesthetic in a community clinic (Fig. 7.5).

Vasectomy is not immediately effective, as sperm can be present in the vas deferens for up for 4 months post-procedure. After 3–4 months, the man will be asked to produce a semen sample for analysis, and will be given the 'all clear' when two samples are seen to be azoospermic, although rules at different centres vary slightly.

POST-VASECTOMY COMPLICATIONS

Post-vasectomy complications are few and are less serious than those for female sterilisation, but should be mentioned. Complications include continued scrotal pain (significant in 8%), infection or haematoma formation at the wound site.

TERMINATION OF PREGNANCY

> **USEFUL WEBSITES**
>
> - British Pregnancy Advisory Service <www.bpas.org>.
>
> - Marie Stopes International, providing choices in reproductive healthcare <www.mariestopes.org.uk>.
>
> - NHS abortion provision <www.nhs.uk/conditions/abortion>.

Approximately 200,000 pregnancies are terminated in the UK each year and this number is constantly rising. The UK abortion services are safe and carry no long-term risks to the woman. This is in stark contrast to abortion services in many other countries, where termination of pregnancy is illegal and performed in unsuitable places using dangerous techniques. Abortion-related deaths account for one-fifth of maternal deaths world-wide.

UK LAW AND INTERNATIONAL LEGISLATION

Termination of pregnancy (TOP) is legal in the UK (but not Northern Ireland) up to the 24th week of a normal pregnancy and up to term for a pregnancy where fetal abnormality has been identified. Currently, in the UK, termination of pregnancy is only allowed if two doctors agree that the circumstance meets one of the listed criteria. Doctors are under no obligation to sign this form, but are obligated to refer the woman to an abortion service if it is her request, and to provide impartial, non-judgemental advice.

The legal criteria the woman must meet to be allowed to terminate their pregnancy are as follows:

- The continuance of the pregnancy would involve risk to the life of the pregnant woman greater than if the pregnancy were terminated.

- The termination is necessary to prevent grave, permanent injury to the physical or mental health of the pregnant woman.

- The pregnancy has not exceeded its 24th week and that the continuance of the pregnancy would involve risk, greater than if the pregnancy were terminated, of injury to the physical or mental health of the pregnant woman.

- The pregnancy has not exceeded its 24th week and that the continuance of the pregnancy would involve risk, greater than if the pregnancy were terminated, of injury to the physical or mental health of any existing child or children of the family of the pregnant woman.

- There is a substantial risk that, if the child were born, it would suffer from such physical or mental abnormalities as to be seriously handicapped.

CHOOSING TO TERMINATE A PREGNANCY

There are a number of reasons why women seek termination of pregnancy and the choice to proceed is rarely easy. Many women require support both before and after an abortion, and it is important that she knows where to access such support. All abortion providers (whether private or NHS funded) provide free counselling before and after their treatment.

The RCOG guidelines recommend that no woman should wait more than 3 weeks from the time of her request to the time of the procedure, and that services should be organised so that they are separate from other gynaecological work.

MEDICAL TERMINATION OF PREGNANCY

Medical termination of pregnancy, also known as the 'abortion pill', is available to women who are less than 9 weeks pregnant. Taking a pill that induces miscarriage is an attractive option to many women, who find surgery embarrassing and invasive.

The first tablet contains 200 mg of Mifepristone an antiprogestogenic steroid (600 mg may also be used), This acts to cut off the hormone supply to the pregnancy, and ripens the cervix. The woman needs to take the tablet at the site of an abortion provider, under medical supervision, and can then go home. She is advised that she may feel slight period-like cramps and experience some vaginal spotting, but is not expected to pass the pregnancy at that point.

The woman will be invited back to the abortion provider 24–48 hours later, to be given the second part of the treatment – four Misoprostol 200 mcg tablets. Centres differ, but the woman can either go home with the advice that cramping pelvic pains and vaginal bleeding will start over the next hour, or can stay to pass the pregnancy in the centre (most centres encourage the first option due to constraints of space and nursing care). Most pregnancies are passed within the first 4 hours of taking Misoprostol, but it can take up to 72 hours. Once the pregnancy is passed, pelvic cramps settle, bleeding reverts to that of a normal period, and settles after a few days.

Absolute contra-indications to medical termination

- Over 35 years of age and smoking more than 10 cigarettes a day.
- Suspected ectopic pregnancy.
- A history of heart disease, high blood pressure, liver or kidney disease.
- Taking long-term corticosteroids.
- IUD in place.
- Adrenal failure.
- Taking anti-coagulants or any haemorrhagic disease.
- Porphyria.
- Poorly controlled inflammatory bowel disease.
- Breast feeding.

After 9 weeks, medical termination is not generally used, but regimens are available.

Effectiveness of medical termination of pregnancy

The medical termination is effective in 98% of cases; to ensure that the 2% in whom the treatment will fail are not missed, women are usually given a pregnancy test to take home and carry out 3 weeks after the abortion. The women found to have a continuing pregnancy, or retained products of conception, will be offered a surgical procedure. However, a pregnancy test can stay positive up to 9 weeks after successful termination of pregnancy.

SURGICAL TERMINATION OF PREGNANCY

Surgical termination of pregnancy is offered to women from the time of confirmed intra-uterine pregnancy up to the 24th week of pregnancy. There are different procedures depending on the gestation. Generally speaking, the smaller the pregnancy, the easier and safer the procedure, but below 7 weeks the failure rate rises and medical methods are generally preferred.

Under 13 weeks' gestation, suction aspiration is generally used. This is safe, quick and effective. It can be carried out without anaesthetic, with local anaesthetic (lignocaine gel), conscious sedation (half-asleep) or general anaesthetic.

Between 13–19 weeks of gestation, dilatation and evacuation is the generally chosen technique, and is usually done under general anaesthetic, unless there is high risk associated with this. Above 19 weeks' gestation, a two-stage procedure is required. The first stage is cervical preparation which involves placement of a mechanical dilator into the cervix and Misoprostol high into the vagina (usually done in the morning). The second stage involves evacuation of the fetus (usually done in the afternoon of the same day). Feticide and induction of labour may be needed for very late procedures.

Rhesus immunisation should be given if the mother is rhesus negative, and chlamydia testing should be offered to all women, whether undergoing the surgical or medical procedure.

It is essential that future contraceptive arrangements are discussed before the procedure so that a suitable method can be started at the time of termination. There is no place for telling the women to wait for her next period to start contraception, she may well have a second unwanted pregnancy if such advice is given.

SUBFERTILITY

USEFUL REFERENCE

- NICE Guidance: Fertility: assessment and treatment for people with fertility problems <http://guidance.nice.org.uk/CG11>.

Subfertility is said to affect up to one in seven couples. It is defined to be the absence of conception after 12 months of unprotected sexual intercourse that has occurred at least twice weekly throughout that period. Approximately 84% of couples will have conceived within a 12-month period; of those who did not conceive, approximately half will go on to conceive spontaneously during the second year of trying.

Couples who are worried about their fertility can become very distressed, and put great pressure on their GP for 'something to be done'. In general, there is no need to investigate or refer until at least a year of trying for a pregnancy has passed; if there are reasons to suspect a problem (such as a history of pelvic infection or an ectopic pregnancy, recurrent miscarriage, irregular or absent cycles, or if the woman is over age 35 years), then referral should be made much sooner. It is helpful if the first investigations are done in primary care, so that specialist appointments are not wasted on basic work.

CAUSES OF SUBFERTILITY

There are a number of causes of subfertility, the most common of which are:

- Male factors.

- Tubal blockage including endometriosis.

- Ovarian dysfunction causing anovulation or infrequent ovulation.

- Structural abnormalities which cause distortion of the uterine cavity.

- Medical problems.

- Immunological factors.

- Maternal age. Female fertility starts to decline after the age of 35 years; with regular intercourse, 94% of women aged 35 years but only 77% of those aged 38 years will conceive after 3 years. The effect of male age is less clear.

It is important that GPs advise all couples who are trying to conceive that they will optimise their chances of success by the cessation of smoking, the avoidance of excessive alcohol, and by achieving an ideal body mass index of 19–30 kg/m^2 (this advice applies to the male as well as the female partner). Regular light exercise, and avoidance of stress also helps conception. The woman should be advised to take folic acid 400 mcg daily. Most pregnancies result from sexual intercourse which occurs in the 5 days preceding ovulation, but the best advice is not for couples to concentrate only on that time, but to try to have regular sexual intercourse about 3 times weekly, throughout the menstrual cycle.

Before any referral is made, both partners should be tested for chlamydia, the woman's immunity to rubella checked and her cervical cytology updated, if necessary.

It is important to ask if there are any difficulties with intercourse. Erectile dysfunction, ejaculatory failure, vaginismus or low libido may not be revealed unless the question is put directly.

MALE FACTORS CAUSING SUBFERTILITY

Male factors account for approximately 40% of couples' subfertility. Such factors include azoospermia or oligospermia, erectile and/or ejaculatory difficulty. It is important that both the male and the female partner are investigated after presenting with subfertility. For the man, this involves collection of a semen sample; this should be collected by masturbation following at least 2 days of sexual abstinence. The semen should be collected in a plastic urinalysis pot, and examined under a microscope within 1 hour of collection. If the gentleman lives some distance from the hospital, he is usually offered the option of producing the sample in a specially designated room within the hospital.

The normal parameters for semen analysis are as follows. An ejaculate should be at least 2 ml in volume, with at least 20 million spermatozoa per millilitre which 50% should be motile and 15% should be of normal morphology. The pH should be over 7.2. There should be less than 1 million leukocytes present per millilitre.

Low semen volume may be due to dysfunction of accessory glands such as the prostate, retrograde ejaculation, or simply difficulty collecting the sample in the analysis bottle. A low sperm count can be idiopathic, or it can be structural such as that due to a blocked vas deferens (e.g. following chlamydial infection, or following vasectomy). It can also be due to a number of behavioural reasons, such as smoking or drug use, or the taking of hot baths. Poor sperm mobility may be a result of infrequent ejaculation, or due to infection.

An abnormal semen analysis should always be repeated, as results can vary over time. It is poor medical practice to give the female partner a bottle and form and ask her to send the man for a sperm count; remember that if it is abnormal the news can be devastating for many men and so informed consent must be given. As such, the male partner must see the GP and request the test himself, and the results are entered on his own medical notes.

Treatment is often by assisted conception, including intracytoplasmic sperm injection (ICSI; sperm retrieval from the testes). For hypogonadotrophic hypogonadism, gonadotrophins may be needed. Chromosome analysis may be indicated for men with hypogonadism.

FEMALE FACTORS CAUSING SUBFERTILITY

Tubal blockage

Tubal blockage and peritoneal adhesions can be caused by pelvic inflammatory disease, endometriosis, or any previous pelvic surgery. A previous ectopic pregnancy may have resulted in salpingectomy, in which case one of the fallopian tubes will be absent.

Assessment of tubal patency is by hysterosalpingography (HSG), which effectively evaluates the patency of the fallopian tubes, as well as revealing any uterine cavity abnormalities. HSG is performed under ultrasound guidance during the follicular phase of the menstrual cycle.

Treatment may be surgical or by assisted conception. There are many techniques for assisted conception, such as intra-uterine insemination, IVF, ICSI, and gamete intra-fallopian transfer (GIFT). None of these offer a 'quick fix' and media stories may distort patients' perceptions of these treatments.

Ovarian dysfunction

Anovulation is another relatively common reason why couples fail to conceive. All women should have blood tests done for FSH on days 2–5 of the menstrual cycle to assess the woman's ovarian reserve. An FSH level greater than 10 IU/ml with an oestradiol level of less than 50 pg/ml indicates decreased ovarian reserve, and an FSH level greater than 20 IU/ml suggests the perimenopause (see Module 6). Whether ovulation is occurring each menstrual cycle can be assessed by taking a serum progesterone level 7 days before the expected next menstruation, i.e. day 21 of a 28-day cycle, or day 23 of a 30-day cycle. A serum progesterone level of 30 ng/ml indicates a successful ovulation and adequate luteal progesterone production. It should be remembered that progesterone is produced by the corpus luteum in tonic pulses in response to the pulses of LH released from the anterior pituitary gland; therefore, a single serum progesterone level should not be relied on if low, but tests should be carried out on three consecutive menstrual cycles before a conclusion is drawn.

If the woman's cycles are regular there is no need to check thyroid function or prolactin, but this should be done if cycles are irregular, long or absent. Remember that antipsychotic drugs may cause hyperprolactinaemia.

Treatment of ovarian dysfunction is that of correcting an underlying disorder should there be one. Women with diabetes mellitus or polycystic ovarian syndrome may benefit from the administration of metformin which can help restore ovulation (this should only be done by specialist centres). Women who are not ovulating due to an eating disorder (e.g. anorexia nervosa or morbid obesity) can restore their ovarian function to normal by achievement of a normal body mass index. Stress, depression, and anxiety can arrest ovulation, and treatment of these often results in restoration of a normal menstrual cycle.

Some women require ovarian stimulants such as clomifene. This should be given in the secondary care environment rather than in primary care, unless instructed to do so by secondary care. This is because clomifene and other ovarian stimulants carry a risk of ovarian hyperstimulation which can be dangerous, and even life-threatening. Clomifene also carries the risk of multiple pregnancy; therefore, close monitoring must be carried out, which may involve ultrasound scanning and monitoring of gonadotrophin levels. The use of gonadotrophins for women who are resistant to clomifene requires special expertise.

Premature ovarian failure needs to be managed by egg donation or surrogate motherhood as appropriate.

Distortion of the uterine cavity

Any cause of uterine cavity distortion can result in subfertility due to difficulty in conception as well as recurrent pregnancy loss. Examples of this include fibroids that project into the uterine cavity or block the fallopian tubes or anomalies of the uterus such as bicornate uterus. Treatment, if possible, is by surgery.

Asherman's syndrome is an uncommon cause of subfertility; it is caused by scarring of the uterine cavity that causes the walls of the uterine cavity to stick together. Asherman's syndrome can result from dilatation and curettage of the uterus, for example, following termination of pregnancy or evacuation of retained products of conception. Asherman's syndrome can usually be corrected by hysteroscopic dissection of the adhesions.

Medical problems

Any chronic medical problems such as diabetes mellitus, thyroid disease, epilepsy, etc. can make conception difficult, particularly if the condition is not diagnosed or poorly controlled. Management of the medical condition can be done by the GP in the usual way, but referral to an obstetrician prior to conception is advised in order to plan the pregnancy and ensure the best possible outcome for the couple and their baby. This advice also applies to all prospective mothers with complex medical conditions who may not have any difficult conceiving (e.g. women with congenital heart disease), who also need their pregnancies to be planned.

NICE recommends that up to three cycles of assisted conception should be available if the woman is aged 23–39 years, and there is an identified case of the failure to conceive (or no cause but no pregnancy after 3 years). However, Primary Care Trusts vary in their willingness to fund this, and it is essential to be familiar with your local guidance and to keep up-to-date on changes.

USEFUL WEBSITE

- Human Fertilisation and Embryology Authority <http://guide.hfea.gov.uk>.

Couples should be counselled carefully before considering private treatment, as a pregnancy is not guaranteed and the cost can be ruinous for people of modest means. The possibility of adoption should not be forgotten.

Module 8:
What's not in the syllabus

Although this chapter contains information that is not requested for the DRCOG examination, the topics discussed below are highly relevant to any doctor working in the field of women's health. Module 8 covers controversial issues which, should you not have come across in work or personal experience as yet, you almost certainly will do so in the near future. Women are often treated differently to men in society; this can be appropriate and necessary, but may be unwelcome, discriminatory and hurtful, causing morbidity, which presents to the GP.

ABUSE OF WOMEN

SEXUAL ABUSE AND RAPE

Some women (as well as some men and children) are, on occasion, subjected to sexual abuse. This can be extremely damaging, both physically and psychologically. Sexual abuse is a term used to describe any forced sexual act. This includes fondling, kissing, photography and other such intimate activities against the individual's will. Rape is the term used for forced penetrative sex (anal or vaginal). Rape can result in the transmission of sexually transmitted diseases including HIV, unwanted pregnancy, loss of virginity, and with loss of virginity comes the loss of social status in many societies. Sexual abuse can lead to long-term problems with confidence, future relationships and self-perception.

In the UK, there are specialised centres that deal with victims of sexual abuse at the time immediately following the assault. They will provide prophylactic drug treatments when indicated, hepatitis B vaccination, emergency contraception, and emotional support. They are also able to document evidence of the assault to assist in prosecution at a later date. A counselling service is available.

PROSTITUTION

Prostitution is said to be the oldest profession. It is that of a woman accepting money from a man who buys the privilege to have sex with her. Many women go into this trade of their own will, but a very large proportion of women are sold into the profession at a young age by family members, or are coerced into it unknowingly perhaps being told they were going to work as a maid in a hotel. Many enter the trade due to their addiction to illicit drugs.

Prostitution is illegal in many countries, but is has always been legal in the UK; a woman is allowed by law to receive money for sex as long as she consents to the deal. However, activities such as pimping (a third person accept-

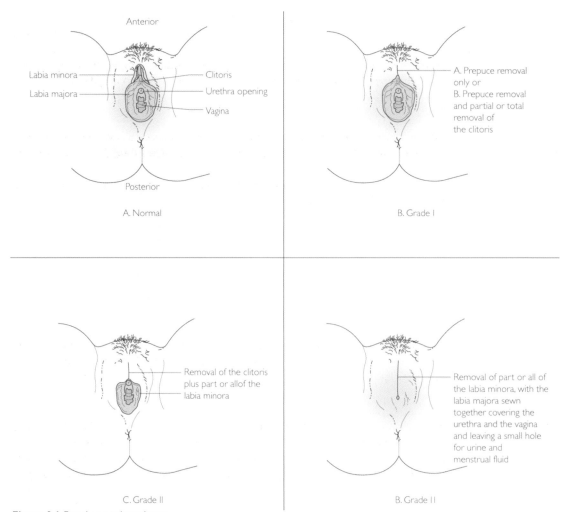

Figure 8.1 Female genital mutilation.

ing money for the activity), running a brothel, kerb-crawling and soliciting are all illegal. Other countries have different laws, some outlawing the trade completely (such as in Pakistan or Russia), whereas in other countries (such as Germany and The Netherlands), prostitution is entirely legal and subject to income tax as with any other job.

Prostitutes are particularly vulnerable to violence from both their customers and intimate partners. They are encouraged to insist on condom usage with customers in order to protect themselves from sexually transmitted infections. Prostitutes are also advised to have regular sexual health check-ups. It is important that they have a reliable, long-term, contraceptive method if they want to avoid pregnancy. They should be vaccinated for hepatitis A and B.

HUMAN TRAFFICKING

Because prostitution is such a successful business, there is often demand for women that out-strips supply. This situation is exacerbated, as customers often prefer younger women to older women. As a result, there is a constant demand for new, young women to enter the trade but, more often than not, young girls are unwilling to go into such an arrangement of their own accord and so are coerced. Typically, the families of women from poor countries are bribed or deceived into letting their daughters go to work far from home, with the promise of food, shelter and a good wage. Once away from their support network, the girls find themselves dependent on their pimp, sometimes addicted to drugs that they were introduced to forcibly, and working as sex-slaves for a number of years. These women have multiple health needs, especially when they fall pregnant. They may carry a number of emotional problems and difficulties with relationships. Financial and social problems may become apparent as they grow older and are rejected by the trade. Human trafficking is illegal in most countries of the world, including the UK.

FEMALE GENITAL MUTILATION

Female genital mutilation (Fig. 8.1), also known as female circumcision or genital cutting, is an extremely wide-spread practice across parts of Africa and the Middle East, and in those immigrant populations throughout the world. The practice is, however, illegal in the UK.

Women who have been mutilated in this way may present to the GP with recurrent urinary tract infections, dyspareunia or psychosexual issues. Child-birth can be difficult.

ETHICAL ISSUES

COSMETIC SURGERY

Women seek cosmetic surgery as a means of fulfilling their emotional needs and resolving problematic body image issues.

Breast augmentation, vulval rejuvenation and facial lifts are typical examples of surgical procedures that are undergone by women, at great financial and personal expense, for no real physical indication. However, societal pressures can be such that a woman feels inadequate in herself, and believes that surgery will help her come closer to achieving what she wants in life, perhaps by boosting her confidence, or making her more lovable by others.

Breast augmentation

The female breasts, being one of the prime symbols of femininity and motherhood and a crucial male attractant, may be viewed as a vital component of female gender identity. If a woman judges her breasts to be 'too small' or 'the wrong shape', she may feel unable to satisfy a man, or her baby. She can, therefore, feel dissatisfied in herself and may suffer from low self-esteem. This, however, is simply a matter of perception, and there is evidence that even after surgical procedures, self-confidence may remain persistently low as other areas of the body are focused on as being inadequate once the breasts have been optimised.

Hymen repair

Hymen repair is a popular operation in the Middle East, particularly in Egypt, where female virginity at the time of marriage is not only highly valued, but is crucial. If the hymen is found to be perforate on the wedding night, it can lead to rejection of the wife and renouncement of the marriage. Due to such intense pressures, women who are unmarried yet known to have a perforated hymen (be that due to forbidden sexual activity, rape, or innocent damage) may seek surgical repair so as not to be embarrassed on their wedding night.

Whether or not doctors should be performing such procedures is debatable, as it is unclear whether such surgery is in the best interest of the women, and wider society or not.

USEFUL WEBSITE

- RCOG statement 2009 opposing hymenoplasty and labial surgery for social or cosmetic reasons <www.rcog.org.uk/files/rcog-corp/Statement6Hymenoplasty.pdf>.

EUGENICS

FETAL SEX DETERMINATION

It is possible to determine the sex of a fetus with reasonable accuracy as early as at 16 weeks' gestation if a good high-resolution ultrasound machine is available. There are a number of cultures and societies that value having a son more than a daughter; this can lead to strong pressure to abort a female fetus. The practice of fetal sex determination and abortion of female fetuses is common in Asia (although illegal), and in India and China the practice has resulted in there now being millions more boys and men in the population than there are girls and women. In China, there are currently approximately 120 male babies born for every 100 female babies according to local data. This leads to a number of social problems, especially when adult males are unable to find wives due to a national shortage.

In the UK, fetal sex determination is allowed and the news is often told to parents at their 20-week anomaly scan. However, abortion is illegal on the grounds of fetal sex.

FETAL SEX SELECTION

Pre-implantation diagnosis can be carried out on viable embryos before implantation following *in vitro* fertilisation (IVF). This provides the opportunity for a huge number of genetic attributes of the fetus to be determined prior to implantation. However, pre-implantation tests are only legal in the UK if performed for medical, rather than social, reasons and the Human Fertilisation and Embryology Authority strictly regulates the tests. Pre-implantation tests are allowed for about 50 genetic conditions, including sickle cell anaemia, Huntingdon's disease, spinal muscular atrophy and cystic fibrosis.

Gender selection prior to implantation is only permissible by law if there is a clear medical indication to do so, such as history of a gender-specific condition. In all other cases, couples undergoing in vitro fertilisation are not allowed to choose the sex of their implanted embryos.

EGG AND SPERM DONATION

There is a great shortage of egg and sperm donors in the UK; some centres have a long waiting list of up to 2 years. This is thought to be because donors are no longer allowed to give their gametes anonymously and are not permitted to accept any payment. Since 2005, donor-conceived children in the UK have had the legal right to trace their biological parents once they reach 18 years of age, and this can be a daunting thought for many would-be donors who may potentially have hundreds of children looking for them in the future. The law was passed as the consensus view was that the child's right to discover their genetic origins outweighed the donor's wish to privacy. As a result, donors now often only agree to donate to specific couples whom they know personally, for example to a close friend or relative. Sperm banks, from which the donation can be used by up to 10 women, are dwindling. Some British couples consider buying eggs or sperm from abroad. This is both legal and anonymous in many countries, which boast a plentiful supply of donors for couples willing to pay, and will provide treatment to lesbian couples, as well as single women. Such countries include Spain, Crete and the Czech Republic.

SURROGATE MOTHERHOOD

Surrogate motherhood is the controversial practice of a woman being paid by a couple to become pregnant, carry the fetus to term, deliver the baby and then give the baby to the paying couple. Breast-feeding services may or may not be required.

Collaborative reproduction in this way carries a number of ethical issues. There is a clear and artificial separation of genetic, gestational and social parentage, and this can be difficult. The surrogate mother may herself have provided the egg (she may have undergone intra-uterine or high vaginal sperm insemination), or may be implanted with an embryo from the donor couple, in cases where the genetic mother is unable to carry a child through pregnancy for a physical reason such as end-organ failure (for example, renal failure requiring dialysis, or congestive cardiac failure), but has normally functioning ovaries from which ova may be harvested. In the first case, the surrogate mother will also be the genetic mother, but she only becomes pregnant on the understanding that she will give the infant up to another couple for rearing, terminating all of her parenting rights at delivery.

As long as the surrogate mother understands and agrees to such an arrangement, society is generally able to accept the practice. Others feel that to use a woman's body in this way is a form of abuse, and hold the view that only women who are vulnerable and desperate would allow themselves to be used in this way.

In the UK, surrogacy is a legal, yet highly restricted, procedure. It cannot be commercial, which makes it illegal to advertise for or as a surrogate, and illegal for an intermediary organisation to broker surrogacy agreements for profit. However, a formal surrogacy agreement can be made that, although not legally enforceable, can be held up in court if it is considered that it is in the best interests of the child.

Under UK law, the woman who carries a child is the legal mother, and her name must go on the birth certificate. The intended parents then need to apply for a parental order that gives them full legal parental responsibility.

List of abbreviations

α-FP, alpha-fetoprotein
ACE, angiotensin-converting enzyme
ACTH, adrenocorticotropic hormone
AIDS, acquired immunodeficiency syndrome
ALT, alanine transaminase
AST, aspartate transaminase

BASHH, British Association for Sexual Health and HIV
Beta-HCG, beta-human chorionic gonadotrophin
BMI, body mass index
BNF, *British National Formulary*
bpm, beats per minute
BSCC, British Society of Clinical Cytologists

CEMACH, Confidential Enquiry into Maternal and Child Health
CIN, cervical intra-epithelial neoplasia
COC, combined oral contraceptive
CT, computed tomography
CTG, cardiotocography

DCCT, Diabetes Control and Complications Trial
DEET, diethyltoluamide
DVT, deep vein thrombosis

ERPC, evacuation of retained products of conception

FBS, fetal blood sampling
FFP, fresh frozen plasma
FSH, follicle stimulating hormone
FSRH, Faculty of Sexual and Reproductive Healthcare (RCOG)

GBS, group B streptococcus
γ-GT, gamma-glutamyl transpeptidase
GIFT, gamete intra-fallopian transfer

GMC, General Medical Council
GnRH, gonadotrophin releasing hormone
GP, general practitioner

HAART, highly active anti-retroviral therapy
hCG, human chorionic gonadotrophin
HELLP, haemolysis, elevated liver enzymes, low platelets
HIV, human immunodeficiency virus
HPV, human papilloma virus
HRT, hormone replacement therapy
HSG, hysterosalpingography
HSV, herpes simplex virus

ICSI, intracytoplasmic sperm injection
IFFC, International Federation of Clinical Chemistry and Laboratory Medicine
IUCD, intra-uterine contraceptive device
IUD, intra-uterine device
IUGR, intra-uterine growth restriction
IUS, intra-uterine system
IVF, *in vitro* fertilisation

LH, luteinizing hormone
LSCS, lower segment caesarean section

MC&S, microscopy, culture and sensitivity
MCV, molluscum contagiosum virus
MMR, measles, mumps, and rubella
MRI, magnetic resonance imaging
MRSA, methicillin-resistant *Staphylococcus aureus*
MSU, mid-stream urine

NAAT, Nucleic Acid Amplification Test
NICE, National Institute for Health and Clinical Excellence
NSAIDs, non-steroidal anti-inflammatory drugs
NSU, non-specific urethritis

OA, occipito-anterior

OAE, oto-acoustic emissions

OP, occipitoposterior

OT, occipitotransverse

PCOS, polycystic ovarian syndrome

PCT, Primary Care Trust

PID, pelvic inflammatory disease.

PMR, perinatal mortality rate

POCT, point of care testing

POP, progesterone-only pill

PPH, postpartum haemorrhage

PROM, premature rupture of membranes

RCOG, Royal College Obstetricians and Gynaecologists

SERM, selective oestrogen receptor modulator

SHBG, sex hormone binding globulin

SIDS, sudden infant death syndrome

SMP, statutory maternity pay

SPP, statutory paternity pay

STIs, sexually transmitted infections

TENS, transcutaneous electrical nerve stimulation

TOP, termination of pregnancy

uE3, unconjugated oestriol

UKMEC, UK Medical Eligibility Criteria

UTI, urinary tract infection

VIN, Vulval intra-epithelial neoplasia

Index

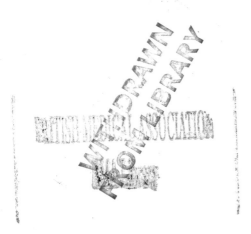